Official Organ of the European Society for Paediatric Endocrinology

Hormone Research

International Journal of Experimental and Clinical Endocrinology

Founded 1970 as 'Hormones' by M. Marois

AF815365

KARGER

Printed in Switzerland
on acid-free paper by
Thür AG Offsetdruck, Pratteln

Appears monthly:
2 volumes per year (12 issues)

Hormone Research

'*Hormone Research*' aims to provide rapid publication of clinical investigations and case reports, as well as experimental and methodological work related to endocrinology. Correspondence is welcome, but publication of letters is at the discretion of the editors.

Submission: Only original papers written in English are considered and should be sent to:

S. Karger AG
Editorial Dept. 'Hormone Research'
P.O. Box
CH-4009 Basel (Switzerland)

Manuscripts should be submitted in triplicate (with three sets of illustrations of which one is an original), typewritten double-spaced on one side of the paper, with a wide margin.

Conditions: All manuscripts are subject to editorial review. Manuscripts are received with the explicit understanding that they are not under simultaneous consideration by any other publication. Submission of an article for publication implies the transfer of the copyright from the author to the publisher upon acceptance. Accepted papers become the permanent property of 'Hormone Research' and may not be reproduced by any means, in whole or in part, without the written consent of the publisher. It is the author's responsibility to obtain permission to reproduce illustrations, tables, etc. from other publications.

Arrangement:
Title page: The first page of each paper should indicate the title (main title underlined), the authors' names, and the institute where the work was conducted. A short title for use as running head as well as the full address of the author to whom correspondence should be sent are also required.
Full address: The exact postal address complete with postal code must be given at the bottom of the title page. Please also supply Phone and Fax numbers.
Key words: For indexing purposes, a list of 3-10 key words in English is essential.
Abstract: Each paper needs an abstract of up to 10 lines.
Small type: Paragraphs which can or must be set in smaller type (case histories, test methods, etc.) should be indicated with a 'p' (petit) in the margin on the left-hand side.
Footnotes: Avoid footnotes. When essential, they are numbered consecutively and typed at the foot of the appropriate page.
Tables and illustrations: Tables and illustrations (both numbered in Arabic numerals) should be prepared on separate sheets. Tables require a heading and figures a legend, also prepared on a separate sheet. For the reproduction of illustrations, only good drawings and original photographs can be accepted; negatives or photocopies cannot be used. When possible, group several illustrations on one block for reproduction (max. size 181 × 223 mm) or provide crop marks. On the back of each illustration, indicate its number, the author's name, and 'top'. Color illustrations are reproduced at the author's expense.
References: In the text identify references by Arabic numerals [in square brackets]. Material submitted for publication but not yet accepted should be noted as 'unpublished data' and not be included in the reference list. The list of references should include only those publications which are cited in the text. Do not alphabetize; number references in the order in which they are first mentioned in the text. The surnames of the authors followed by initials should be given. There should be no punctuation other than a comma to separate the authors. Cite all authors, 'et al' is not sufficient. Abbreviate journal names according to the Index Medicus system. (Also see International Committee of Medical Journal Editors: Uniform requirements for manuscripts submitted to biomedical journals. Br Med J 1988;296: 401-405.)
Examples
(a) Papers published in periodicals: Kauffman HF, van der Heide S, Beaumont F, Blok H, de Vries K: Class-specific antibody determination against *Aspergillus fumigatus* by means of the enzyme-linked immunosorbent assay. III. Comparative study: IgG, IgA, IgM ELISA titers, precipitating antibodies and IgE binding after fractionation of the antigen. Int Arch Allergy Appl Immunol 1986;80:300-306.
(b) Monographs: Matthews DE, Farewell VT: Using and Understanding Medical Statistics. Basel, Karger, 1985.
(c) Edited books: Hardy WD Jr, Essex M: FeLV-induced feline acquired immune deficiency syndrome: A model for human AIDS;in Klein E (ed): Acquired Immunodeficiency Syndrome. Prog Allergy. Basel, Karger, 1986, vol 37, pp 353-376.
Further details: Authors may consult our leaflet 'Rules for the Preparation of Manuscripts', available on request from the Publisher, S. Karger AG, P.O. Box, CH-4009 Basel (Switzerland).

Page charges: There is no page charge for papers of 4 or fewer printed pages (including tables, illustrations and references). Each additional complete or partial page is charged to the author at SFr. 415.-/ US$ 275.00. The allotted size of a paper is equal to approx. 12 manuscript pages (including tables, illustrations and references). As the page charges are waived in any case for the first paper each year to be published by a member of ESPE, authors who are members of the ESPE should so indicate on the title page.

Galley proofs: Unless indicated otherwise, galley proofs are sent to the first-named author and should be returned with the least possible delay. Alterations made in galley proofs, other than the correction of printer's errors, are charged to the author. No page proofs are supplied.

Reprints: Order forms and a price list are sent with the galley proofs. Orders submitted after the issue is printed are subject to considerably higher prices. Allow five weeks from date of publication for delivery of reprints.

KARGER

General Information

Hormone Research

Publication data: 'Hormone Research' is published 12 times annually. Volumes 39–40 with 6 issues each appear in 1993

Subscription rates: Subscriptions run for a full calendar year. Prices are given per volume.

Personal subscription:

Subscription + postage and handling
SFr. 278.60 + SFr. 16.80 Europe
SFr. 278.60 + SFr. 25.20 Overseas
US$ 186.20 + US$ 16.80
(Must be in the name of, billed to, and paid by an individual. Order must be marked 'personal subscription'.)

Institutional subscription:

Subscription + postage and handling
SFr. 398.– + SFr. 24.– Europe
SFr. 398.– + SFr. 36.– Overseas
US$ 266.00 + US$ 24.00

Airmail postage: SFr. 36.–, US$ 30.00. (Extra per volume.)

Discount subscription prices:
European Society of Paediatric Endocrinology. Lawson Wilkins Society; ISGD; Schweizerische Gesellschaft für Endokrinologie.

Microform edition: SFr. 199.–, US$ 133.00. (Available exclusively to subscribers of the paper edition.)

Subscription orders: Orders can be placed at agencies, bookstores, directly with the Publisher S. Karger AG, P.O. Box, CH – 4009 Basel (Switzerland) or with any of the following distributors:

Deutschland: S. Karger GmbH
Lörracher Strasse 16A, Postfach
D-W-7800 Freiburg

France: Librairie Luginbühl
36, bd de Latour-Maubourg, F-75007 Paris

Great Britain, Ireland: S. Karger Publishers
11 Ravenscroft Road
Beckenham, Kent BR3 4TP

USA: S. Karger Publishers, Inc.
26 West Avon Road, P.O. Box 529
Farmington, CT 06085

India, Bangladesh, Sri Lanka:
S. Karger India Subscription Agency
B – 5/132 Safdarjung Enclave
New Delhi-110029

Japan: Katakura Libri, Inc.
36-9 Hongo 3-chome, Bunkyo-ku, Tokyo 113

Change of address: Both old and new address should be sent to the subscription source.

Single issues and back volumes: Information can be obtained through the Publisher.

Advertising: Correspondence and rate requests should be addressed to the Publisher.

Bibliographic indices: This journal is regularly listed in bibliographic services, including *Current Contents®*.

Book Reviews: Books are accepted for review by special agreement.

Guidelines for Disk Submission

Karger Publishers welcomes the submission of manuscripts on disk.

Please observe the 'Instructions to authors' as well as the following guidelines:

Technical Data

The preferred **storage medium** is a 3.5- or 5.25-inch disk in MS-DOS format. Macintosh is also acceptable.

The preferred **word processing package** is Microsoft Word. Other commonly used PC text programs are also accepted, as well as ASCII formats.

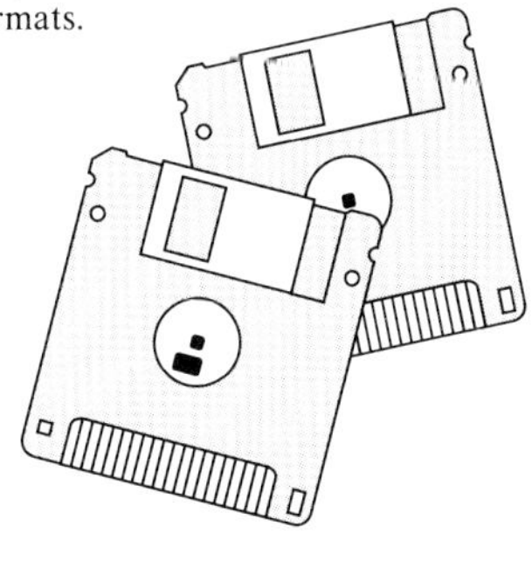

Handling

All manuscripts accepted for Karger publications are subject to copy editing. It is therefore essential that you send us a **double-spaced printout** of your manuscript which exactly matches the disk.

Any subsequent revised versions should be clearly marked as such, both on the disk and on the manuscript.

The copy-edited manuscript and the disk will be returned to you along with the galley proofs. Please be sure to **check the galleys against the manuscript** in which changes introduced by the copy editor and/or questions will be marked.

Please **label** your disk with (a) the title of the journal for which it is submitted, (b) a short version of the paper title, (c) your name and (d) the software and hardware used.

Text Arrangement

Text and headings should be ranged left throughout, without word breaks. **Do not center, space, or use block letters** for text and headings (except for abbreviations).

Do not use indentations to mark the beginning of a paragraph, but use one blank line between paragraphs.

Be sure to use the **same type style for headings of the same ranking** throughout the text.

When using **special characters** not available on a standard keyboard (including Greek characters), please do so by a readily identifiable code, and use the same code throughout the manuscript. Supply a **complete list of the codes used** at the beginning of the text.

Illustrations, tables and mathematical formulae will be handled conventionally.

KARGER

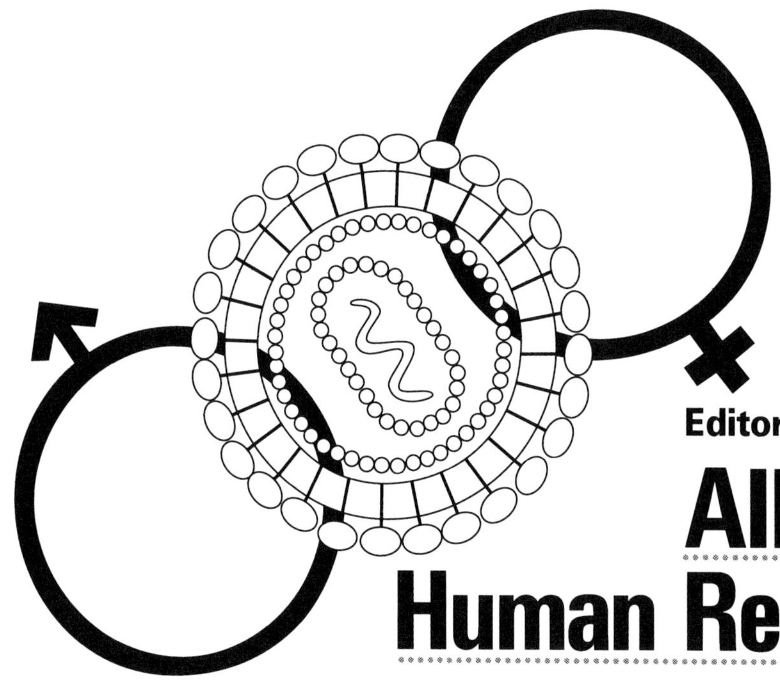

Aging of Reproductive Organs

Aging of Reproductive Organs

First Tokyo Conference on
Reproductive Physiology II
Tokyo
August 22, 1992

Guest Editors
Y. Taketani, Tokyo
S. Kawagoe, Yamagata

23 figures, 5 tables, 2 color plates, 1993

KARGER

Hormone Research

Vol. 39, Supplement 1, 1993

S. Karger
Medical and Scientific Publishers
Basel · Freiburg · Paris · London
New York · New Delhi · Bangkok
Singapore · Tokyo · Sydney

Drug Dosage
The authors and the publisher have exerted every effort to ensure that drug selection and dosage set forth in this text are in accord with current recommendations and practice at the time of publication. However, in view of ongoing research, changes in government regulations, and the constant flow of information relating to drug therapy and drug reactions, the reader is urged to check the package insert for each drug for any change in indications and dosage and for added warnings and precautions. This is particularly important when the recommended agent is a new and/or infrequently employed drug.

P.O. Box, CH-4009 Basel (Switzerland)
Printed in Switzerland on acid-free paper by
Thür AG Offsetdruck, Pratteln
ISBN 3-8055-5797-3

Contents

Horm Res 1993;39 (suppl 1):1

Preface

T. Aso
S. Kawagoe
A. Miyake
H. Mori
Y. Nakamura
Y. Taketani

With the advent of a longevous world, research on aging has received great impetus. We, gynecologists, are dealing with reproductive phenomena which seem to be contrastive to aging phenomena. Indeed, aging is, in a narrow sense, an age-related decrement of functions in cells, tissues, organs, or the whole body, finally leading to individual death. However, it is of interest to think that aging is a time-dependent imbalance of homeostasis. In other words, aging can be interpreted as alterations of a wide variety of functions by distorting homeostasis and thereby causing changes in developmental or functional state during individual life. In that sense, reproductive phenomena in which drastic changes of morphology and functions take place, appear to be analogous to aging.

With this in mind, we think the time is just right to review aging for better understanding reproductive physiology. Thus, we discussed various aspects of aging in connection with reproduction at the Tokyo Conference on Reproductive Physiology II held on the 22nd August 1992, and compiled the contents herein.

The members of the organizing board would like to thank all the participants of the conference for their active and constructive discussions which made the conference a great success. We would also like to extend our appreciation to Japan Sandoz Co. Ltd., whose sponsorship enabled us to hold the conference and publish this supplementary issue.

Organizing Board
(in alphabetical order)

Takeshi Aso
Department of Obstetrics and Gynecology
Tokyo Medical and Dental University
Tokyo (Japan)

Sinnosuke Kawagoe
Department of Obstetrics and Gynecology
Yamagata University
Yamagata (Japan)

Akira Miyake
Department of Obstetrics and Gynecology
Osaka University
Osaka (Japan)

Hiroyuki Mori
Department of Obstetrics and Gynecology
Teikyo University
Tokyo (Japan)

Yukio Nakamura
Department of Obstetrics and Gynecology
Kyorin University
Tokyo (Japan)

Yuji Taketani
Department of Obstetrics and Gynecology
Tokyo University
Tokyo (Japan)

Horm Res 1993;39(suppl 1):3–4

Shinnosuke Kawagoe

Department of Obstetrics and Gynecology,
Yamagata University School of Medicine,
Yamagata, Japan

The Aging Process of the Reproductive Organs: An Overview

Life is the continuum of a process known as aging, which begins in utero and terminates in death, as if to be born is to start to die. The aging process is accompanied by progressive and irreversible changes in whole organisms. In 1981, Green [1], a gerontologist, defined aging as 'a progressive deterioration of the organism after maturity of size, form, or function has been reached and which is universal, intrinsic, progressive, and deleterious with time.' These aging changes involve the degeneration of most, if not all, tissues and organs, decline in functional capacity of physiological systems, and loss of function in homeostatic mechanisms between and within organs and systems. Although many important advances in the physiopathological interpretation of the aging phenomena in humans and animals were made in the past, fundamental questions remain unanswered. What are the nature or central causes of age-related physiologic deterioration?

Several different but probably related hypotheses have been advanced to be responsible for aging. As an example, 'programmed death' or 'gene regulation' theory has been proposed; i.e., the aging processes are basically progressed according to a program prearranged inheritantly. This hypothesis is based primarily on the findings that the maximum life-span varies considerably from one species of animal to another and appears to be specifically fixed at a certain length in each species or even in the strain of these species. It is conceivable that undoubtedly many factors are at work to place limitations on one's life-span. Some of these factors, such as the capacity for cell repair or renewal, may be genetically determined. With the wane of optimum function of the repair systems, cellular aging starts. The process of mitosis or cell division may be slowed down or fall into abeyance.

In conjunction with this hypothesis, another one is so-called 'error catastrophe' or 'molecular injury' theory. In the cells exposed to a certain level of physical and chemical stimuli, damage to DNA may occur, which may in turn result in an accumulation of metabolic errors within the cells during their life-span. If the repair systems are inefficient, unrepaired damage in DNA will increase relatively rapidly. As these errors accumulate, cells are interfered significantly with their substantial function and stop cycling ultimately due to DNA damage.

There is now sufficient evidence, most of it recent, showing that free radical reactions which can be initiated by many chemical and physical agents may be strongly related to cellular mechanisms of aging processes. For example, lipid peroxidaton in vivo has been identified as a basic deteriorative reaction to lead to cell damage. Furthermore, it has been shown that the specific activity of superoxide dismutase (SOD), which is a major protective enzyme against oxygen toxicity, of the tissue or of the whole adult organism is positively correlated with maximum life-span potential for all the primate species. This correlation strongly suggests that longer-lived species have a higher degree of protection against by-products of oxygen metabolism [2]. Although living organisms do contain many physiological free radicals, there are several known factors, such as SOD, and probably others unknown at this time, that can protect susceptible biomolecules from the uncontrolled radical reactions. Thus, along with the decrease in the capacity for preventing radical mechanisms during the process of aging, unrepaired cellular damage may occur, and consequently, these damages may result in loss of functional capacities of physiological systems. However, consideration should also be given to

Shinnosuke Kawagoe, MD
Department of Obstetrics and Gynecology
Yamagata University School of Medicine
2-2-2 Iida-Nishi, Yamagata 990-23 (Japan)

0301–0163/93/0397–0003
$2.75/0

factors that alter the activities of antioxidants and radical scavengers in preventing damage.

There is no question that age changes affecting reproductive capacity occur in several organs in aged females of all mammalian species. Regardless of our lack of better understanding of the mechanisms involved in the aging processes, age-related physiologic deterioration of the human ovary is of special interest. It appears more convincing to conclude that the neuroendocrine system is mainly responsible for the aging process of the ovary. It is also evident, however, that the ovary may autonomically lose its own function, because ovarian failure occurs relatively rapidly with increasing age in spite of continued hypothalamo-pituitary stimulus. While most endocrine functions are modified only slightly and slowly during the life of the individual, ovarian function seems to be an exception. The functional decline and loss of the aging ovary begin so early and occur even more precipitously. Aging changes in both structure and function of the ovary in mammalian species have been well documented so far. In the human female, structural changes in aged ovary are generally characterized by a striking diminution of primordial follicles and increase in amount of connective tissue. At the time of menopause, only a small number of follicles remain, but these no longer respond to gonadotropic hormones. Thus, ovarian steroid production in women approaching the menopause decreases dramatically in spite of increased gonadotropin output by the hypophysis. These investigations provide indirect support to the concept of Longscope [3] that the intrinsic mechanism of the menopause is an alteration of ovarian sensitivity to gonadotropins. The causes of reproductive decline associated with increasing maternal age is thought primarily to be the result of ovarian failure. What, then, are the mechanisms behind such dramatic changes in menopausal ovaries?

In this issue, possible mechanisms for the age-related changes in body processes will be reviewed first, and the aging of the ovaries will be discussed from the histological and biochemical viewpoints. Furthermore, there is no doubt that, in addition to the age changes in the ovary, aging of both the ova and the uterus is another important factor in the decline in reproductive capacity. The delay in ovulation or in fertilization may probably play a significant role in abnormal embryonic development and aneuploidy, and as a consequence increased loss of the conceptus may be more likely to occur. Although these pathogeneses have not been clearly understood in the human female, some data supporting such a possibility will be presented in this issue. In addition, the biochemical changes occurring in the uterus with age, which appears to be the primary cause of reproductive failure in some species, will also be discussed.

References

1 Green M: Aging and disease. Clin Endocrinol Metab 1981;10:207–228.
2 Tolmasoff JM, et al.: Superoxide dismutase: correlation with life-span and specific metabolic rate in primate species. Proc Natl Acad Sci USA 1980;77:2777–2781.
3 Longscope C: Steroid production in pre- and postmenopausal women; in Greenblatt RB (ed.): The Menopausal Syndrome. New York, Medcom Press, 1974.

Horm Res 1993;39(suppl 1):5–8

K. Suzuki

Department of Molecular Biology,
School of Medicine, Tokai University,
Isehara, Kanagawa, Japan

Origin of Senescence: A Review

Key Words
Life-span gene
Longevity gene
Oxygen free radicals
Nematode
Oxygen-sensitive mutant

Abstract
The aging process is controlled by dual mechanisms. One is the mechanism which programs ultimate cell death and therefore determines the life-span at birth. The other is the mechanism which causes aging stochastically by damaging certain substances with time in life. Now, these mechanisms have been investigated on genetical bases. Whatever the mechanisms involved in aging, increasing evidence suggests the important roles of oxygen free radicals in the process of aging.

Introduction

In the search of mechanisms of aging, a variety of theories have been postulated. The studies of aging have been achieved based upon various levels, such as molecular, cellular, organ, or whole body, etc. It is generally difficult to describe ubiquitous mechanisms of aging. For example, if immunological events are taken up as an example for potential causes of certain aging phenomena, the changes are finally manifested as a decrease in the number of immune cells. The decrease in these cells may be derived from a decrease in the number of bone marrow stem cells which might be caused by the aging process in DNA levels. One may wonder what mechanisms are involved in the changes at DNA levels. In this review, the author attempts to explore the ultimate cause of aging which underlies at the initial level of the chain of events leading to the apparent aging phenomena. Especially, several problems to be considered in fundamental aging research will be described.

Are Changes with Aging a Cause or Result of Aging?

It is generally very difficult to clarify whether observed changes with aging are causes or results of aging. The misunderstanding concerning this issue can be found in various studies dealing with aging, for instance, comparison between young and old persons or comparison between long-lived and short-lived animals. Therefore, these comparative studies seem to be of limited value. Recently, aging studies based on genetical analyses are considered promising to evade the above-mentioned confusion. Namely, genes controlling the aging process or life span are currently being investigated in lower animals such as the nematode. The identification of homologous genes in the human being will open a new dimension in the study of human aging. In addition, the transgenic animal model into which the gene involved in aging is incorporated may be instrumental in understanding the aging mechanisms.

K. Suzuki, MD
Department of Molecular Biology
Tokai University School of Medicine
Isehara, Kanagawa 259-11 (Japan)

0301-0163/93/0397-0005
$2.75/0

Dual Control of Aging

It is evident that aging or longevity of animals is eventually controlled by genes. Table 1 summarizes thus far presented notions of the aging mechanisms at genetic level. One of the genes called *the life-span gene* is to determine life-span by regulating the aging process and thereby programming ultimate cell death. This notion came from the observation by Hayflick and Moorehead [1] that growing cells have a limited number of doubling. It is also known that doubling the number of human diploid cells reduces with advanced age of the donor. Cells obtained from patients with Werner's syndrome, a disease characterized by premature aging, show a lower number of doubling compared with cells from normal control at a corresponding age [2]. Dominant expression of certain substances which may accelerate the aging process has been shown in experimental animals by Tauchi [3] and in human diploid cells by Fujiwara [pers. commun.]. Recently, programmed cell death was investigated on a genetic basis in the developing nematode, *Caenorhabditis elegans*, by Ellis et al. [4]. This study proposed the following genes involved in systemic cell death: the gene which determines cells to be killed; the gene which is involved in killing; the gene concerning engulfing and pyknotic cell killing by surrounding cells, and the gene for degradation of killed cells.

The other gene for regulating aging is *the longevity gene* which seems to assure longevity of species and have reproductive cycles completed. Individuals after finishing reproduction have no significant 'raison d'être' for certain populations and reasonably accept senescence possibly caused by endogenous and exogenous environmental factors such as oxygen free radicals, radiations, etc. The existence of some genes is proposed which protect cells from these unfavorable factors. The concept of senescence determined by a balance between attacking factors and protective factors was postulated as the 'wear-and-tear theory' by Medvedev [5] and Orgel [6]. A recent study by Cutler [7] elegantly demonstrated that the scavenging capability of oxygen free radicals correlated well with the maximal life expectancy in various primates, including humans. A mutant of *Drosophila* which is completely defective in the activity of Cu/Zn superoxide dismutase has a very short life-span (10 days' half-life), by far shorter compared with that of the wild-type (60 days) [8]. Likewise, a mutant of nematode, *C. elegans*, with low activity of the enzyme also has a shorter life-span than that of the wild-type [9].

Table 1. Dual gene functions for aging

The life-span gene	The gene which programs the process of aging (senescence) and eventually determines lifespan
The longevity gene	The gene which controls the mechanism to tolerate endogenous and exogenous environmental factors leading to senescence

Table 2. Cellular types and estimated mechanism for cell death

Cell type	Cell death
Nondividing nonregenerative type	
Neuron, heart muscle, nephron, alveoli, liver (?)	Spontaneous death by oxygen-related free radicals Programmed death in some cases (e.g. neurons in development)
Nondividing regnerative type	
Blood cells	Spontaneous death as above Decrease in regenerating cells
Ever-dividing cells	
Epithelial cells of small intestine and skin, fibroblasts, bone marrow stem cells	Spontaneous death as above Programmed death in some cases (e.g. fibroblasts)

Complexity in Understanding Aging

In discussing aging, the process of senescence is often intermixed with longevity. It should be kept in mind that longevity is controlled by the onset of the senescence process and its progression rate. These two aspects should be taken into consideration separately in understanding aging. Furthermore, several lines of mechanisms have been postulated at cellular level as shown in table 2. However, these mechanisms cannot be applied ubiquitously since some proper mechanisms may work in rapidly growing bone marrow cells or undividing nerve cells. At any rate, whatever the mechanisms of aging, it appears that the onset of senescence and its process are associated with a decrease in number of cells in question.

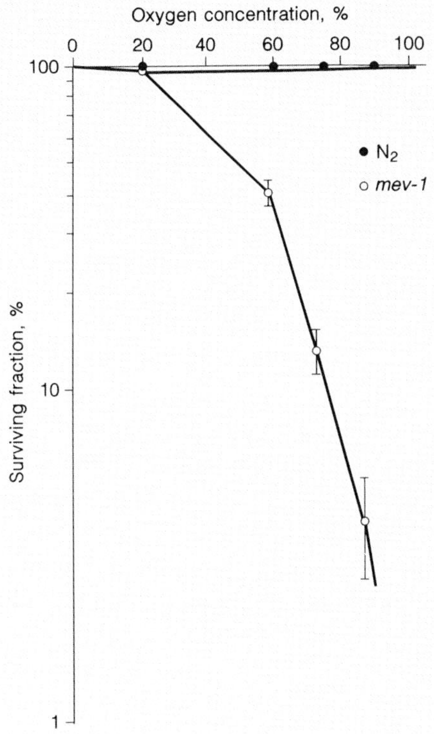

1

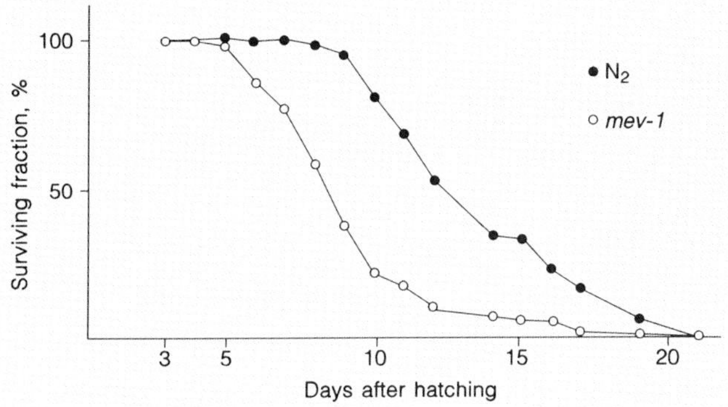

2

Fig. 1. *mev-1* mutant of *C. elegans* is highly sensitive to gaseous oxygen. L_1 larvae of both wild-type (N2) and *mev-1* were exposed to O_2/N_2 at various concentration ratios and survival was determined after 3 days. Vertical bars are standard deviation derived from four repeated experiments in which about 100 animals were used for one experiment.

Fig. 2. *mev-1* mutant has a shorter life-span as compared with that of the wild-type. About 100 animals were observed for one experiment. Animals were cultivated at 20 °C on agar plates with *Escherichia coli* strain OP50 as food. Survivals were scored at the days indicated in the figure.

Oxygen Free Radicals as Possible Etiological Factors for Aging

Since oxygen free radicals are now widely known to be a pathogenic factor for a variety of diseases [10], it is reasonable to speculate that they are also involved in aging which occurs in any part of the body. Oxygen free radicals are always generated by the mechanisms whereby our lives are maintained. Thus, it may be that aging is an unavoidable process as long as we live. In our recent study using the nematode, *C. elegans*, a mutant form, *mev-1*, was isolated which is highly sensitive to both gaseous oxygen and methyl viologen (paraquat) [9] as shown in figure 1. Genetic analysis revealed that the mutation is located on chromosome 3. The average life-span of the mutant is 9.4 days, still shorter than that of the wild-type (14.3 days) as depicted in figure 2. The short life-span of the mutant may be attributed to decreased levels of Cu/Zn superoxide dismutase activity, with one-half activity of the wild-type. One common chromosomal abnormality, monosomy-21, is associated with a relatively short life. Reduction in the enzyme activity was also reported in this case by Nakai et al. [11].

Conclusion

The aging process can be considered to be caused by a decrease in the number of cells in tissues or organs. Since the whole body is composed of different types of cells, a decrease in cell number or cell death may be conducted in various manners depending on the locations or sorts of cells. Although a single mechanism of aging was recently proposed, such as the melatonin theory [12], dual mechanisms controlling aging stated here do not contradict it. At any rate, free radicals are emphasized as possible decisive factors in modulating the aging process.

References

1 Hayflick L, Moorehead PS: The serial cultivation of human diploid cell strains. Exp Cell Res 1961;25:585.

2 Nikaido O, Ban S, Sugahara T: Population doubling number in cells with genetic disorder; in Okada K (ed): Aging Phenomena. New York, Plenum Press, 1978, pp 303–311.

3 Tauchi H: Studies of aging with parabiosis; in Oota (ed): Gerontology (in Japanese). Tokyo, Asakura Book Co, 1976 pp 145–160.

4 Ellis RE, Yuan J, Horwitz HR: Mechanisms and functions of cell death. Annu Rev Cell Biol 1991;7:663–698.

5 Medvedev ZH: Repetition of molecular genetic information as a possible factor in evolutionary changes in life span. Exp Gerontol 1972;7:227.

6 Orgel LE: Aging of clones of mammalian cells. Nature 1973;243:441.

7 Cutler RG: Free radicals and aging; in Roy AK, Chatterjee B (eds): Molecular Basis of Aging. New York, Academic Press, 1984, pp 263–354.

8 Phillips JP, Campbell SD, Michaud D, Charabonneau M, Hilliker AJ: Null mutation of copper/zinc superoxide dismutase in Drosophila confers hypersensitivity to paraquat and reduced longevity. Proc Natl Acad Sci USA 1989;86:2761–2765.

9 Ishii N, Takahashi K, Tomita S, Keino T, Honnda S, Yoshino K, Suzuki K: A methyl viologen-sensitive mutant of the nematode *Caenorhabditis elegans.* Mutat Res 1990;237:165–171.

10 Southorn PA, Posis G: Free radicals in medicine. II. Involvement in human diseases. Mayo Clin Proc 1988;63:390–408.

11 Nakai H, Kada K, Abe Y: Erythrocyte superoxide dismutase-1 and 21-trisomy. Cytogenet Cell Genet 1984;37:547.

12 Armstrong SM, Redman F: Melatonin: A chronobiotic with anti-aging properties. Med Hypotheses 1991;34:300–309.

Horm Res 1993;39(suppl 1):9–15

Tatsuo Shimada[a]
Tetsuo Morita[a]
Kaoruko Nagai[a]
Fuminori Sato[a]
Hiroyuki Mori[b]
Gordon R. Campbell[c]

[a] Department of Anatomy, Oita Medical University, Oita,
[b] Department of Obstetrics and Gynecology, Teikyo University, Tokyo, Japan;
[c] Department of Anatomy, University of Queensland, Brisbane, Qld., Australia

Morphological Changes in Spiral Artery of the Mammalian Ovary with Age

Key Words
Aging
Spiral artery
Ovary, human and monkey
Morphology

Abstract
Morphological changes which take place in ovarian arteries at different ages in human and monkey, were investigated by light microscopy, transmission electron microscopy and scanning electron microscopy. The ovarian arteries in both species were characterized by a spiral configuration throughout their course. The hilar and medullar arteries were especially convoluted. In the pubertal monkey, the hilar and medullary arteries exhibited some intimal thickenings in which smooth muscle cells of a synthetic phenotype were longitudinally arranged. These arteries in adult monkeys had considerable intimal thickening. In a 30-year-old woman, arteries with intimal thickenings were detected in the hilus and medulla. Around 40 years of age, the intima of the arteries were considerably thickened with a diameter usually equal to half of the wall. In women after menopause, the tunica intima of these arteries was approximately two-thirds or more of the total artery wall thickness. Spiral arteries of the ovary were also thickened with advancing age.

Introduction

During the twenty-first century, Japanese postmenopausal women will comprise an ever-increasing percentage of the population. What determines the age at which the menopause occurs? Ginsburg [1] concluded that the most important factor determining a woman's age at the menopause is the number of ovarian follicles. The aging of the ovary is marked by a diminution in the number of follicles, which leads to a reduction of circulating inhibin and increased serum FSH [2–4]. As a rule, in mammalian ovaries, more than 99% of the follicles present at birth are destined to degenerate during life [5–8]. Why the great majority of follicles degenerate at various stages of development is not known. Therefore, to date, most studies on aging of the ovary have concentrated on the morphological appearance of follicles and on hormonal aspects. The aim of the present study is to provide some morphological information on aging of the ovarian arteries.

The ovary is well known to have a rich vascularity to facilitate follicular growth, the secretion of steroid hormones and its sensitivity to hormonal agents [9–11]. In 1987, Takada et al. [12] examined spiral arteries in the monkey ovary by scanning electron microscopy (SEM) using vascular casts. Spiral and convoluted configurations of the ovarian arteries in the adult monkey were found by

Tatsuo Shimada
Department of Anatomy
Oita Medical University
Oita 879-55 (Japan)

0301–0163/93/0397–0009
$2.75/0

them to be fundamentally similar to those of human [9, 13]. However, a few reports have been published indicating degeneration of arteries in the ovary of postmenopausal women [9, 14] and adult pigs [15]. In addition, it is noteworthy that ischemia or transplantation leads to the degeneration of a large number of oocytes [6].

This paper therefore uses light microscopy of selectively stained sections, immunohistochemistry, transmission electron microscopy (TEM) and SEM to examine the morphological changes which take place in the arteries of the human and monkey ovary with advancing age.

Materials and Methods

TEM of Monkey Ovarian Arteries

The ovaries of 5 Japanese monkeys, ranging in age from 3 to 12 years, were utilized for this study. The animals were anesthetized with sodium pentobarbital (25 mg/kg), and the ovaries removed. Tissue blocks were immersed in Karnovsky's fixative and postfixed in cacodylate-buffered 2% osmium tetroxide. They were then dehydrated in a graded series of ethanol and embedded in epoxy resin. Thin sections were stained with tannic acid and lead citrate, and examined under TEM. As a control, the femoral arteries were also taken and studied simultaneously.

SEM of Monkey Ovarian Arteries

Four adult femal Japanese monkeys (6–8 years of age) were used. Under anesthesia, ovaries were perfused through the ovarian arteries with a saline solution followed by Karnovsky's fixative. The ovaries were then removed and cut into small pieces with a razor blade. The tissues were placed in the same fixative, postfixed in osmium tetroxide, dehydrated and dried by the *t*-butylalcohol freezing method. Vascular casts of ovarian arteries and branches were prepared according to the Mercox injection method of Takada et al. [12]. All specimens were coated with gold and examined under SEM.

Histology and Immunohistochemistry of Human Ovarian Arteries

The ovaries of 10 patients, ranging in age from 30 to 68 years, which had been removed surgically for treatment of cervical cancer, but without any obvious ovarian disease, were used. Tissue blocks were fixed in 10% formalin solution, dehydrated and embedded in paraffin. Thick sections (6 µm) were stained with a series of techniques: Verhoeff hematoxylin, orange G and phosphomolybic acid-anilin blue (HOPA) staining, silver impregnation techniques (Bielschowsky-Gomori method) and alcian blue (pH 1.0) staining. For immunohistochemistry, 6-µm sections were prepared by the immunogold-silver method [16]. Briefly, the sections were treated with mouse-anti-actin antibody (Zymed), mouse anti-chondroitin-4-sulfate antibody, mouse anti-chondroitin-6-sulfate antibody or dermatan sulfate proteoglycan antibody (Life Science) for 2 h at room temperature. They were then incubated with goat anti-mouse 5 nm gold conjugate (Janssen, N.J., USA) for 1 h at room temperature. Finally, the sections were physically developed for 40 min at 20 °C. All specimens were examined by light microscopy.

As a control, the testes, which had been removed from 53- to 72-year-old men for treatment of prostate cancer, were also studied histologically. Tissue blocks were fixed in 10% formalin and paraffin sections were stained with HOPA.

Result

Structure of the Monkey Ovarian Artery

The monkey ovarian arteries arise from the abdominal aorta just caudal to the origin of the renal arteries. They pass downward, enter the pelvis and reach the ovary via the mesovarium. In both pubertal (3–4 years) and adult (6–10 years) monkeys, the initial one-fifth of the ovarian artery is relatively straight, but the remainder is very tortuous or tightly spiralled. The ovarian arteries are closely associated with the utero-ovarian vein throughout the vascular system.

SEM observations of vascular casts demonstrated that the spiralled portion of the artery was located among the two or three channels of the ovarian vein (fig. 1a). The profuse arterial branches in the hilus and medulla were especially convoluted and had more spiral configurations (fig. 1b). These vessels ran in a spiralling course up to the follicles of the cortex. Under higher magnification SEM, the axes of endothelial cells of the spiral arteries appeared to run parallel to the blood flow (fig. 1b). The cells were usually elongated and regularly arranged (fig. 2a). They were, however, irregular in shape and at the curve and the bifurcation were sometimes damaged (fig. 2b). Lymphocytes and monocytes were also sometimes attached (fig. 2c).

TEM observations of the ovarian arteries and branches revealed significant changes with age. At 3 years of age, spiral arteries in the hilus and medulla showed a normal appearance (fig. 3a). Beneath the endothelium was an

Fig. 1. Scanning electron micrographs of the vascular casts of the adult monkey ovary. **a** A spiral artery (A) running into the pelvis is closely associated with utero-ovarian veins (V). × 7. **b** Spiral arteries in the hilus (H) and the medulla (M) are greatly convoluted. × 35. Inset shows a higher magnification view of a spiral artery. × 100.

Fig. 2. Scanning electron micrographs of the luminal surface of hilar spiral arteries in the monkey. **a** Vessels are tortuous and their endothelial cells run along the course of the vessle. Areas in rectangle are enlarged. × 100. **b** The endothelial cells are irregular in shape and appear to be damaged at the curve. × 1,000. **c** A lymphocyte is attached to the endothelium. × 3,800.

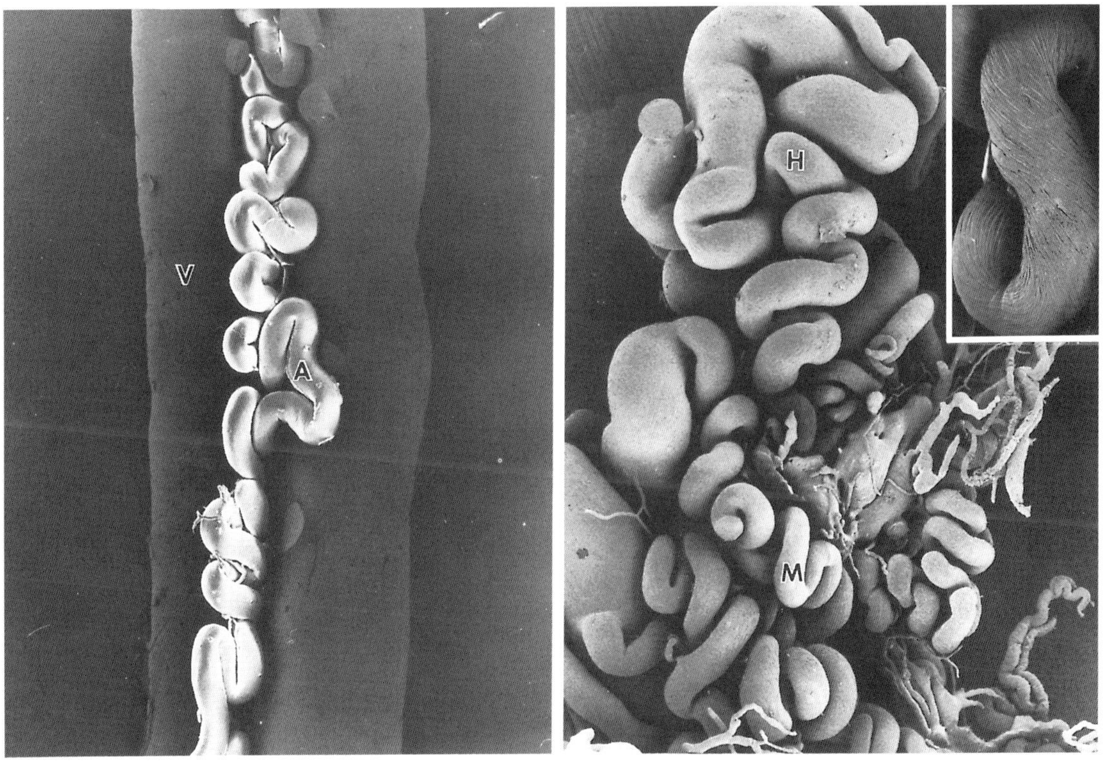

1a 1b

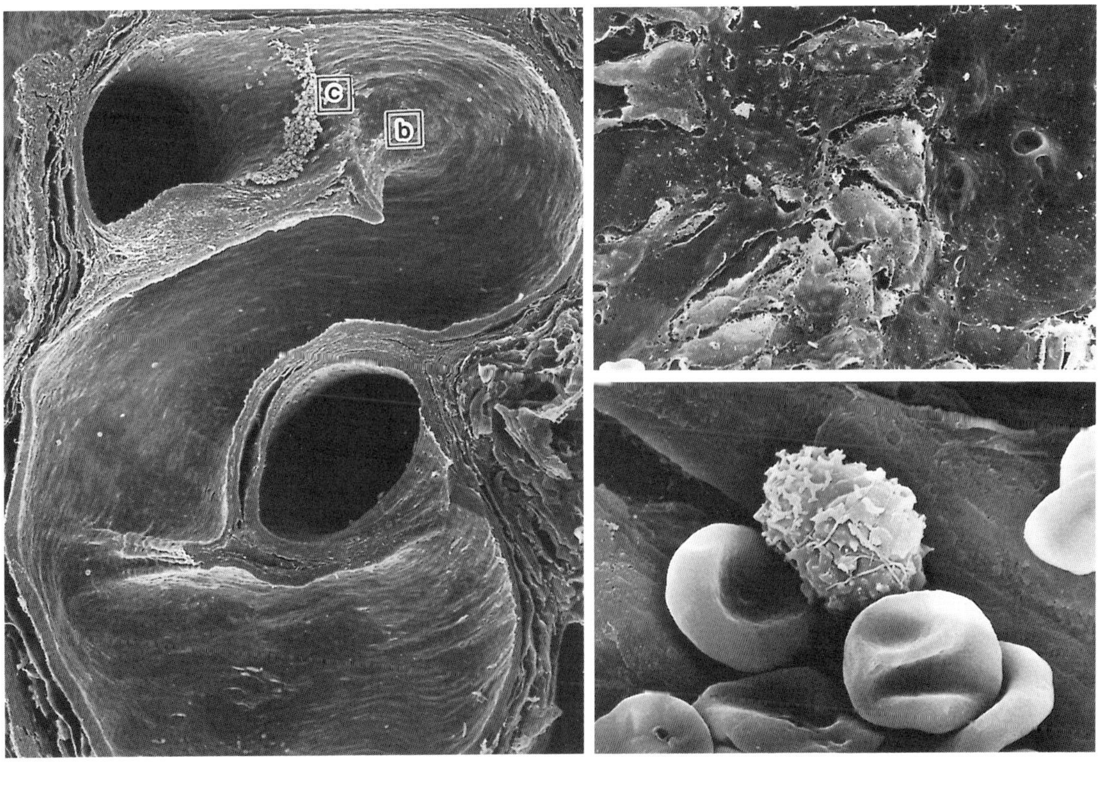

2a 2b 2c

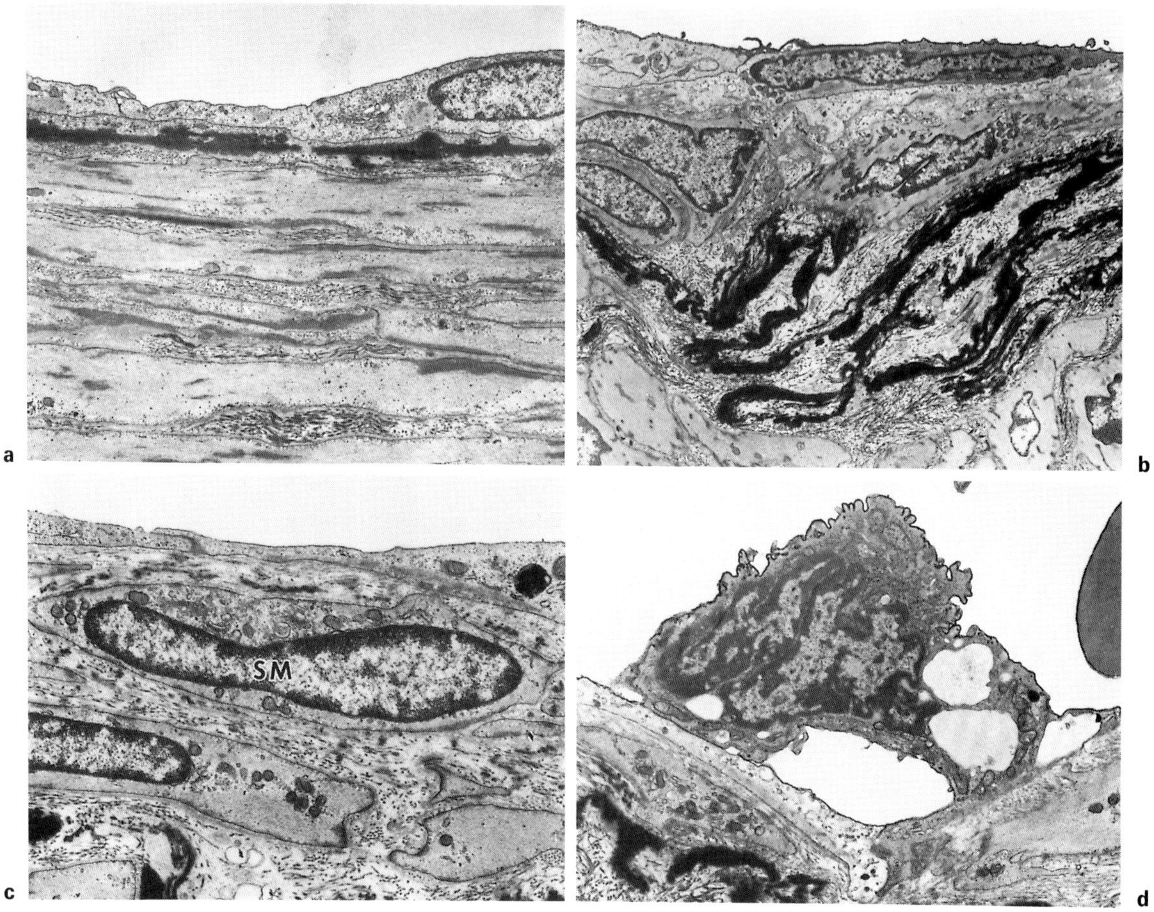

Fig. 3. Transmission electron micrographs of the hilar arteries in the pubertal monkey ovary. **a** At 3 years of age, an artery exhibits a normal appearance, and a single layer of the internal elastic lamina is situated beneath the endothelium. × 5,100. **b** At 4 years of age, an artery shows a thickened tunica intima. Note that the internal elastic lamina is split. × 4,000. **c** A smooth muscle cell (SM), which contains relatively developed cell organelles and small bundles of actin filaments, is present in the thickened intima. × 6,800. **d** In an affected artery, a lymphocyte is attached to the endothelium. × 4,600.

internal elastic lamina consisting of a single layer of elastic fibers. The tunica media of these arteries was composed of approximately 4–5 layers of smooth muscle cells arranged in a circumferential manner. Adrenergic and cholinergic nerves were in close contact with the peripheral smooth muscle cells. At 4 years of age, some spiral arteries in the hilus exhibited a diffuse thickened tunica intima (fig. 3b). This tunica intima contained polygonal-shaped smooth muscle cells, which were arranged longitudinally and possessed large amounts of rough endoplasmic reticulum, Golgi apparatus and small actin filament bundles (fig. 3c). Collagen fibrils and elastic fibers were loosely distributed around these cells. Splitting of the internal elastic lamina was also noticed, and some smooth muscle cells were also present between the split layers. In some arteries, lymphocytes were attached to the endothelium (fig. 3d). At 8–12 years of age, spiral arteries in the same region showed a considerable thickening of the tunica intima (fig. 4a). This tunica intima contained numerous smooth muscle cells and large amounts of fibrous elements such as collagen and elastic fibers. The tunica intima of the hilar arteries was thickened with advancing age. By contrast, most of the femoral arteries in pubertal and adult monkey had a similar appearance (fig. 4b) to that observed in normal mouse femoral artery [17] and human testicular arteries [18].

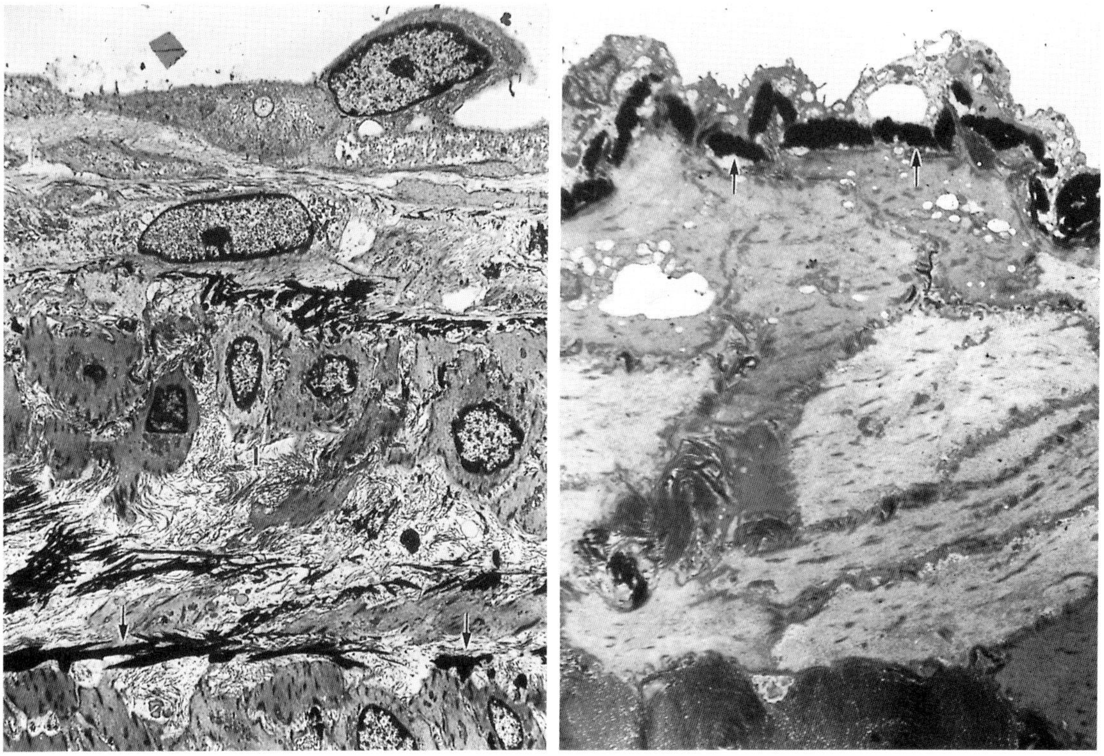

a b

Fig. 4. Ovarian (**a**) and femoral arteries (**b**) of an 8-year-old monkey. Arrows show the internal elastic lamina. **a** The tunica intima (I) of the hilar artery is considerably thickened, possessing numerous smooth muscle cells and large amounts of collagen and elastic fibers. × 1,800. **b** The femoral artery appears to be intact. × 2,600.

Morphological Changes of Arteries in Human Ovarian Tissues

In sections of human ovary stained with HOPA, structures were differentially stained as follows: smooth muscle cells, deep orange; collagen fibers, blue; elastic fibers, dark violet. In ovarian tissues from a 30-year-old woman, a few spiral arteries in the hilus and medulla showed a normal appearance, but most exhibited a thickened tunica intima and splitting of the internal elastic lamina (fig. 5a). In the 38- to 43-year-old group, arteries in both the hilus and medulla showed a considerable thickening of the tunica intima (fig. 5b). This thickening was usually equal to half the whole wall, and contained a large number of polygonal-shaped cells. In the 59- to 64-year-old group, all women from which ovaries were obtained had reached menopause. Few or no follicles were found. The intimal thickening of both the hilar and medullary arteries was approximately two-thirds or more of the entire arterial wall thickness (fig. 5c). Consequently, the lumen of these vessels was greatly reduced. By contrast, in 53- to 72-year-old human testes, spermatogenesis still continues and Leydig cells were observed. The arteries in the tunica albuginea and the mediastinum testis only occasionally had a slightly thickened intima (fig. 5d).

In paraffin sections from human ovary immunogold-silver stained for actin (fig. 6a), intensely positive reactions were found in smooth muscle cells of the media but also in polygonal-shaped cells of the intima. In silver-impregnated sections, the thickened intima was stained a black color (fig. 6b), indicating the presence of large amounts of reticular fibers. In contrast, collagen fibers, which stained a brownish color, were distributed throughout the media and adventitia (fig. 6b).

The thickened intima of affected arteries was heavily stained a blue color (fig. 7a) with alcian blue (pH 1.0) which stains specifically sulfate groups such as chondroitin sulfate proteoglycan [19], indicating that the extracellular matrix of the thickened intima was rich in sulfate groups. In addition, immunohistochemical studies revealed that the matrix of the thickened intima contained chondroitin-6-sulfate (fig. 7b).

Discussion

The ovarian arteries of the human and monkey are characterized by spiral configurations throughout their length [9, 12, 13]. It has been suggested that the spirals in the ovarian arteries are an adaptation of the vasculature to ovarian growth and they provide a mechanism for the reduction and regulation of ovarian blood pressure [12, 13]. In addition, the extensive contact between the veins and arteries is known to provide a mechanism for exchange of heat, gases and other substances [20–22]. Testosterone, progesterone and estradiol are transferred from the utero-ovarian vein into the ovarian artery in the pig [22, 23]. Also, the mature follicles and the corpus luteum have dense networks of blood capillaries because they require a large blood supply [11, 12]. Thus, it is clear that the vascular system of the ovary greatly influences its function.

The number of oocytes in the mammalian ovary varies with age. Some of the oocytes present at birth undergo maturation and ovulate, but most of them become atretic. Postmenopausal ovaries contain very few or no oocytes. By contrast, the human testis still maintains both reproductive and steroidogenic capacities even in old age. Mammalian testicular arteries run in a spiral within the spermatic cord, but arterial branches in the mediastinum testis and in the intralobular connective tissue are straight [24]. In the present histological study, arteries in the testes of 53 to 72-year-old men showed an intact appearance with a slightly thickened tunica intima. Spiral arteries of ovaries in climacteric and postmenopausal women exhibited an extremely thickened intima. The marked intimal thickness of spiral arteries is also present in older sows [15] and Japanese monkeys [present study]. The age when ovarian arteries first demonstrated an intimal thickening, varied in different animal species. It appears to be 22 years in humans [14], 4 years in monkey [present study] and 6 months in the sow [15]. Intimal thickenings in ovarian arteries commence at a young age and increase with advancing age.

In the present study, intimal thickening was most marked in the hilar and medullary arteries of the ovary, but femoral arteries and intratesticular arteries, which run in a straight path, generally displayed no thickenings. Why does this thickening of the tunical intima occur in the ovarian artery? McMillan [25] has suggested that arterial areas exposed to unusually low shear stress, i.e., stagnation regions, are areas most predisposed to atherosclerosis. From a rheological point of view, it is likely that the tightly spiralled arteries in the ovarian hilus and medulla have many low shear stress regions. In SEM observations of the luminal surfaces of monkey spiral arteries, mechanically damaged endothelial cells were often detected. Furthermore, TEM observations of these vessels demonstrated numerous smooth muscle cells not only within the thickened intima but also between the split layers of the internal elastic lamina. The response-to-injury hypothesis as described by Ross [26] would suggest that the endothelium of the ovarian arteries could be injured and growth factors released from endothelial cells and smooth muscle cells. This would then stimulate migration of smooth muscle cells from the media into the intima, and their subsequent proliferation.

The climacteric, which is the transitional period from reproductive to nonreproductive status, is characterized by a marked diminution in the number of follicles and a decrease of estrogen levels [3–5, 13, 27]. There is further evidence that oocytes are very sensitive to ischemia [6, 28]. It has been reported that blood flow to the noncycling ovary is reduced dramatically when compared to the normal cycling ovary [29]. In our histological and immunohistological study, the intraovarian arteries in the climacteric exhibited thickening of the tunica intima and these intimal thickenings were further enlarged after menopause. The intimal smooth muscle cells were of a synthetic phenotype [30] and surrounded by numerous reticular fibers, elastic fibers and proteoglycans. In general, reticular fibers consisted of type I and type III collagens [31]. A number of studies have indicated that estrogen affects the phenotype of smooth muscle and produces an increase in synthesis of extracellular matrix components

Fig. 5. Light micrographs of human ovarian (**a–c**) and testicular (**d**) tissues stained with HOPA. ×150. **a** An artery in the medulla of the ovary of a 30-year-old female shows a thickened tunica intima. **b** At 38 years of age, the intimal thickening of the medullary artery is equal to half the whole wall. **c** At 59 years of age, the lumen of the medullary artery is greatly reduced. **d** An intratesticular artery of a 68-year-old man appears to be intact.

Fig. 6. Light micrographs of arteries in the hilus (**a**) and medulla (**b**) of the ovary of a 59-year-old woman. ×150. **a** In a section immunostained for actin, intensely positive resections are found in cells of both the intima and media. **b** In a silver-impregnated section, the thickened intima is stained a black color, while the media and adventitia are stained a brownish color.

Fig. 7. Light micrographs of arteries in the medulla of the ovary of a 50-year-old woman. ×150. **a** The thickened intima of an affected artery is heavily stained a blue color with alcian blue. **b** In a section immunostained for the chondroitin-6-sulfate, intensely positive reactions are found in the thickened intima.

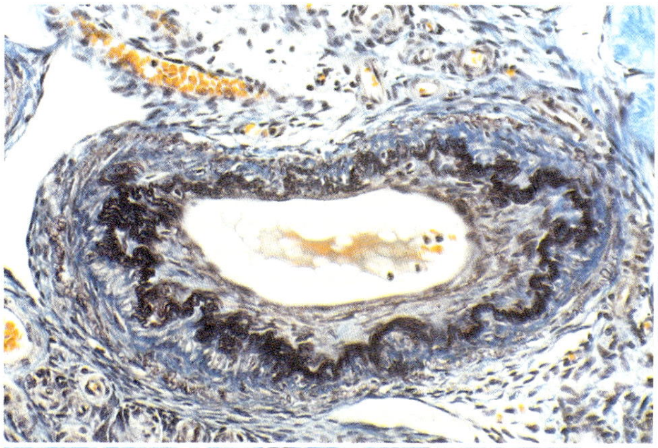
5a

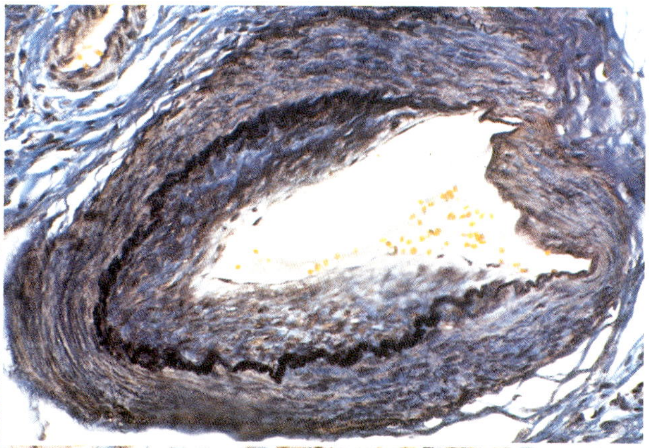
5b

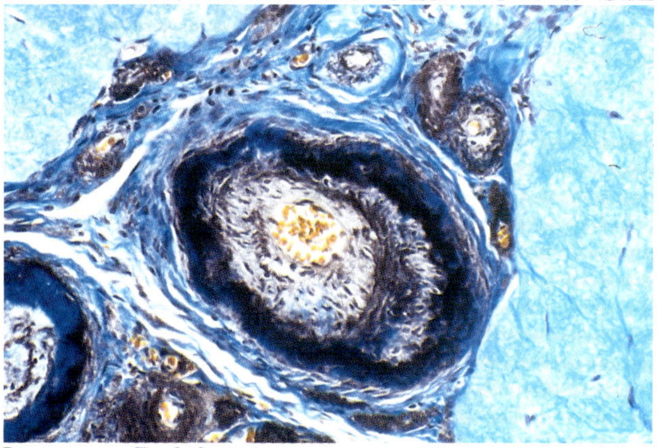
5c

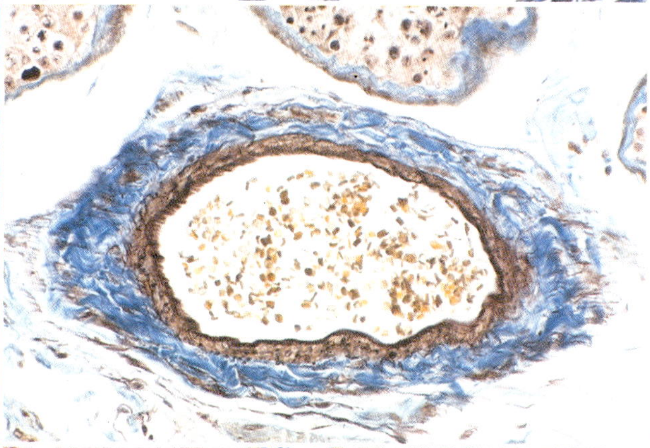
5d

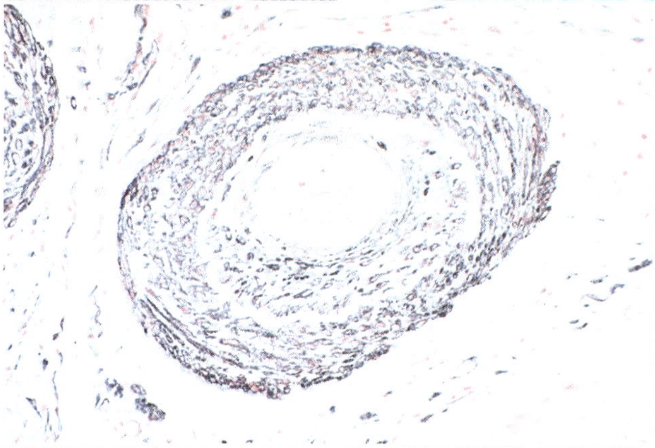
6a

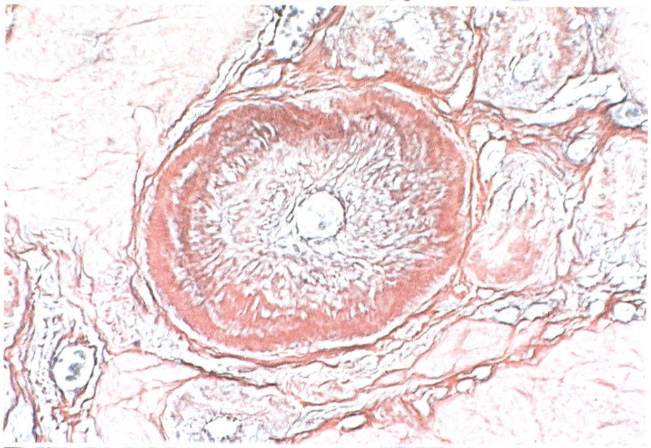
6b

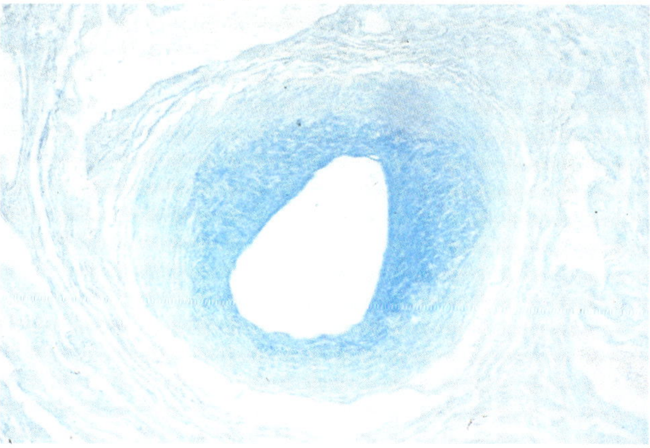
7a

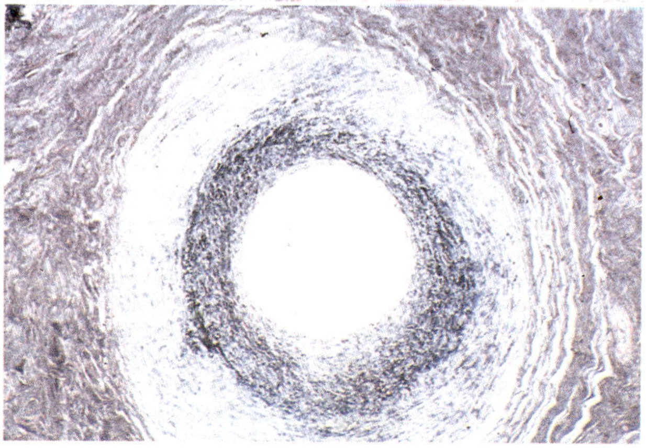
7b

[32–35]. Concentrations of estrogen and progesterone in the pig ovarian artery were significantly higher than other arteries [23].

In conclusion, changes which occur with age in ovarian arteries may influence the ovary. Further studies will be necessary to substantiate this thesis.

Acknowledgments

We thank Dr. Hirokazu Kitamura, Dr. Shin-ichi Takada, Mr. Shuji Tatsukawa and Miss Yukari Goto for encouraging this study. We are also grateful to Prof. Michiaki Yakushiji from Kurume University for access to tissue specimens.

References

1 Ginsburg J: What determines the age at the menopause? The number of ovarian follicles seems the most important factor. BMJ 1991; 302:1288–1289.

2 Mornex R: Physiopathologie de la ménopause. Rev Fr Gynécol Obstét 1985;80:187–190.

3 Utian WH: Overview on menopause. Am J Obstet Gynecol 1987;156:1280–1283.

4 Vagenakis AG: Endocrine aspects of menopause. Clin Rheumatol 1989;8(suppl): 48–51.

5 Block E, Magnusson G, Odeblad E: A study of normal and atretic follicles with autoradiography. Acta Obstet Gynecol Scand 1953;32:1–6.

6 Ingram DL: Atresia; in Zuckerman SS (ed): The Ovary. New York, Academic Press, 1962, pp 247–273.

7 Hertig AT, Barton BR: Fine structure of mammalian oocytes and ova; in Greep RO, Astword EB (eds): Handbook of Physiology, Sect 7, vol II, Part 1. Washington, American Physiological Society, 1973, pp 317–348.

8 Tardif SD: Histologic evidence for age-related differences in ovarian function in tamarins. Biol Reprod 1985;33:993–1000.

9 Clark JG: The origin, development and degeneration of the blood vessels of the human ovary. Johns Hopkins Hosp Rep 1900;9:593–676.

10 Reynolds SRM: The vasculature of the ovary and ovarian function. Recent Prog Horm Res 1950;5:65–100.

11 Burr JH, Davies JI: The vascular system of the rabbit ovary and its relationship to ovulation. Anat Rec 1951;3:273–296.

12 Takada S, Shimada T, Nakamura M, Mori H, Kigawa T: Vascular pattern of the mammalian ovary with special reference to the three-dimensional architecture of the spiral artery. Arch Histol Jpn 1987;50:407–418.

13 Delson B, Lubin S, Reynolds SRM: Vascular patterns in the human ovary. Am J Obstet Gynecol 1949;57:842–853.

14 Kyuragi H: Morphological study about arterial aging process of female genital tract. J Kurume Med Assoc 1978;41:325–340.

15 Bal HS, Getty R: Morphological changes in the vasculature of the ovaries of the sow as influenced by age from birth to 8 years. J Reprod Fertil 1970;22:311–320.

16 Takita K, Shimada T, Kitamura H, Fujii S, Nakamura M: Studies on the physical developer for use in immunohistochemistry. Acta Histochem Cytochem 1990;23:647–662.

17 Rhodin JAG: Fine structure of vascular walls in mammals with special reference to smooth muscle component. Physiol Rev 1962;42:48–87.

18 Fawcett DW: The fine structure of capillaries, arterioles and small arteries; in Reynolds SRM, Zweifach BW (eds): The Microcirculation. Urbana, University of Illinois Press, 1959, pp 1–27.

19 Lev R, Spicer SS: Specific staining of sulfate groups with alcian blue at low pH. J Histochem Cytochem 1964;12:309.

20 Ginther OJ, Dierschke DJ, Walsh SW, Campo CHD: Anatomy of arteries and veins of uterus and ovaries in rhesus monkeys. Biol Reprod 1974;11:205–219.

21 Bendz A, Hansson HA, Svendsen P, Wiqvist N: On the extensive contact between veins and arteries in the human ovarian pedicle. Acta Physiol Scand 1982;115:179–182.

22 Krzymowski T, Kotwica J, Stefanczyk S, Debek J, Czarnocki J: Steroid transfer from the ovarian vein to the ovarian artery in the sow. J Reprod Fertil 1982;65:451–456.

23 Kotwica J, Krzymowski T, Stefanczyk S, Nowicka R, Debek J, Czarnocki J, Kuznia S: Steroid concentrating mechanism in the sow's ovarian vascular pedicle. Adv Physiol Sci 1981;20:149–152.

24 Harrison RG, Weiner JS: Vascular patterns of the mammalian testis and their functional significance. J Exp Biol 1949;26:304–316.

25 McMillan DE: Effects of insulin of physical factors. Metabolism 1985;34:70–77.

26 Ross R: The pathogenesis of atherosclerosis – An update. N Engl J Med 1986;314:488–500.

27 Steger RW, Peluso JJ: Sex hormones in the aging female. Endocrinol Metab Clin 1987;16: 1027–1043.

28 Butcher EO: Regeneration in ligated ovaries and transplanted ovarian fragments of the white rat. Anat Rec 1932;54:87–104.

29 Ellinwood WE, Nett TM, Niswender GD: Ovarian vasculature; in Zuckerman SS (ed): The Ovary. New York, Academic Press, 1962, pp 583–614.

30 Campbell GR, Campbell JH: Recent advances in molecular pathology: Smooth muscle cell phenotypic changes in arterial wall homeostasis. Exp Mol Pathol 1985;42:139–162.

31 Morita T, Shimada T, Kitamura H, Nakamura M: Demonstration of connective tissue sheaths surrounding working myocardial cells and Purkinje cells of the sheep moderator band. Arch Histol Cytol 1991;54:539–550.

32 Albert EN, Pease DC: An electron microscopic study of uterine arteries during pregnancy. Am J Anat 1968;123:165–194.

33 Friederici HHR, Cloux RJ: The early response of immature rat myometrium to estrogenic stimulation. J Ultrastruct Res 1968;22:402–412.

34 Gostimirovich D: Effects of different doses of estrogen on the aortic wall of young immature rabbits. Virchows Arch [A] 1970;349:93–97.

35 Ross R, Klebanoff SJ: Fine structural changes in uterine smooth muscle and fibroblasts in response to estrogen. J Cell Biol 1967;32:155–167.

Horm Res 1993;39(suppl 1):16–21

N. Suganuma
T. Kitagawa
A. Nawa
Y. Tomoda

Department of Obstetrics and Gynecology,
Nagoya University School of Medicine,
Nagoya, Japan

Human Ovarian Aging and Mitochondrial DNA Deletion

Key Words
Aging
Menopause
Human ovary
Primordial follicle
Mitochondrial DNA
Polymerase chain reaction
DNA deletion

Abstract
The functions of human ovary change dynamically around the menopausal period. A decrease of the number of primordial follicles and an increase of fibrous tissues are observed histologically in the aged ovary. As endocrinological aspects at menopause, the synthesis and secretion of ovarian steroid hormones such as estrogens and progesterone decrease, followed with the resultant increases of pituitary gonadotropins. However, the mechanism of menopause and ovarian aging is not well understood. Thus, to study the regulatory mechanism of ovarian dysfunction by aging, we analyzed the accumulation of mitochondrial DNA (mtDNA) mutation in the human ovary in women of various ages. The amplification of a 5.5-kb region in mtDNA with polymerase chain reaction revealed a 0.5-kb band in ovarian samples obtained from menopausal and postmenopausal women, which means that the 5.0-kb deletion of mtDNA in ovarian tissue starts at the menopausal period. The close relationship between the occurrence of ovarian mtDNA deletion and the menstrual irregularity was also observed. These observations suggest that the accumulation of the deleted mtDNA may be a regulating factor of dysfunction of the ovary by aging.

'Aging' is the most universal process of life physiology in all living things. Through reproduction, genetical information of a species is repeatedly transferred to its descendants. The aged individuals' organs and cells diminish in function before their lives finally end.

Among various organs, the ovary seems exceptional in that its function is dramatically curtailed before the completion of the typical life-span of the individual. Organic and functional alterations in the human ovary occur within a very short interval, and the period is called 'menopause'. Menopause indicates the final menstrual period, and occurs during the climacteric that is the phase in the aging process of women that marks the transition from the reproductive stage of life to the nonreproductive stage [1]. Although the essential aspects of the menopause imply the depletion of germ cells and the deficiency of estrogen, the mechanism of the onset of menopause is not clarified. What component in the hypothalamic-pituitary-ovarian-uterine axis is the primer effector of reproductive senescence? What determines the age when menopause starts? Why does the ovary decrease its activity earlier and more completely than the other organs which age gradually?

In this article, we review human ovarian aging at histological and endocrinological sites, and the mechanism of the ovarian senescence in relation to the accumulation of mitochondrial DNA (mtDNA) mutation in the human aged ovaries.

Nobuhiko Suganuma, MD
Department of Obstetrics and Gynecology
Nagoya University School of Medicine
65 Tsurumai-cho, Showa-ku
Nagoya 466 (Japan)

0301–0163/93/0397–0016
$2.75/0

a b

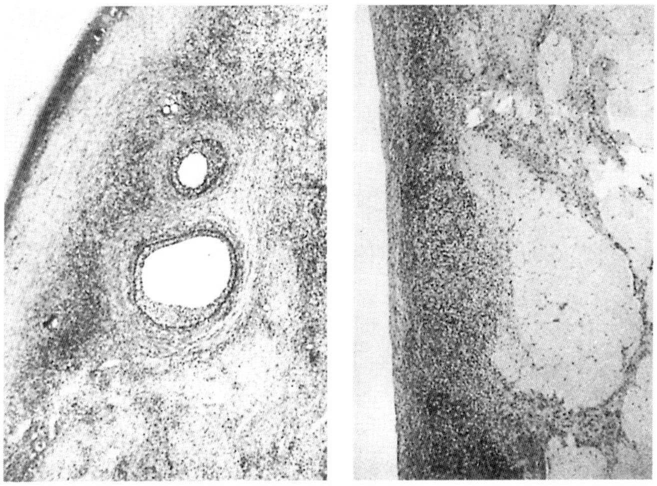

Fig. 1. Human ovaries at the (**a**) reproductive stage (38 years old) and (**b**) postmenopause (60 years old). Although follicles and thick cortex are observed in the younger ovary, the elder one showed the increases of corpus albicans and fibrous tissues, and no primordial follicles. ×100.

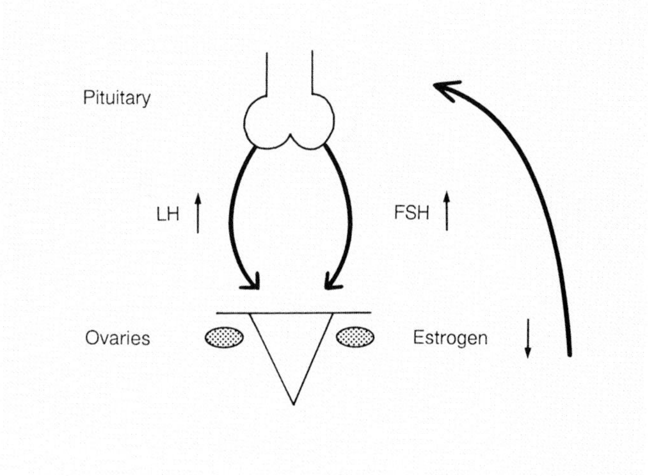

Fig. 2. Scheme of endocrinological characteristics in the menopausal women. The decrease of ovarian estrogen induces the increases of pituitary gonadotropins.

Histological Changes in Human Ovary by Aging

Throughout the reproductive period, the ovary is a dynamic organ that may change its size, shape, and weight at each stage of menstrual phases [2]. After menopause, there is a gradual reduction in ovarian weight to approximately half of the premenopausal ovary [3–5]. In the postmenopausal women, it is clear that the ovary itself ages, resulting in histological changes such as a thickening of blood vessel walls, a gradual disappearance of primordial ova and follicles, and a generalized fibrosis (fig. 1) [6]. Ovarian stromal cells remain to a variable extent and occasionally become hyperplastic [6, 7].

Of 7 million oocytes formed by midgestation, only 2 million are present at birth, and only about 300,000 at menarche [8–10]. Oocyte loss occurs at a constant logarithmic rate during the reproductive years [8], and an accelerated oocyte depletion is observed as menopause approaches [11]. The menopause is undoubtedly due to failing ovarian function due to the exhaustion of the pool of primary follicles, and the associated decreased steroidogenesis.

As mentioned above, the ovaries of approximately one-third of all aging women show hyperthecosis of ovarian stroma cells, indicating continued steroidogenic function [12–16].

Endocrinological Characteristics at Menopausal Period

As women approach menopause, the menstrual cycles become irregular and then ultimately terminate [17]. When menstrual cycles are no longer observed, the women is considered to be menopausal. Menopause is associated with almost a complete loss of oocytes and both an alteration and decline of steroidogenesis within the ovary. The negative feedback effects of estrogen and progesterone to pituitary-hypothalamus are lost, causing an elevation of pituitary FSH and LH, and perhaps an increase in hypothalamic GnRH (fig. 2) [18–20].

Although the menopausal ovary may be lacking in follicles, the cells of which normally secrete estrogen and progesterone, most menopausal women are not totally devoid of estrogen [16, 21, 22]. The ovarian stroma cells have steroidogenic capacity for producing androstenedione, which is converted in peripheral tissues to estrone [23].

mtDNA Mutation in Human Aged Ovary

Mitochondria and Their Own DNA

Mitochondria [24–27] are oval-shaped organelles, and several hundreds to thousands of mitochondria exist in the cytoplasm of all kinds of cells. Electron microscopic

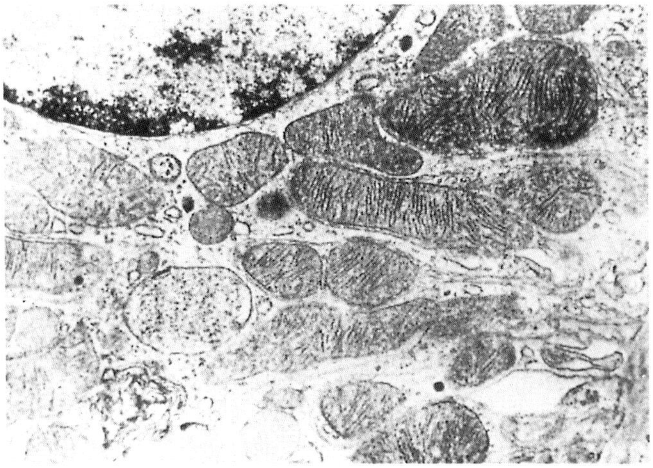

Fig. 3. Electron microscopic feature of mitochondria. A lot of mitochondria exist in the cytoplasm of the cell, and two membranes of mitochondria are observed. [Photograph provided by Dr. Hanaichi, Nagoya University School of Medicine.]

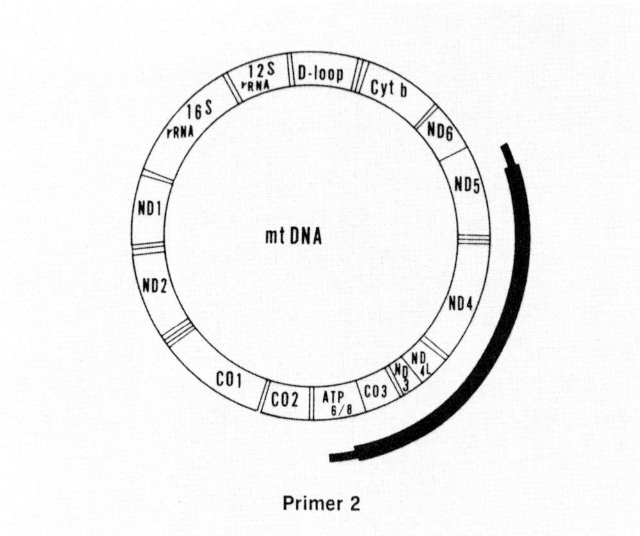

Fig. 4. The physical map of human mtDNA. The primer positions used for the PCR and the amplified part in figure 5 were indicated.

studies revealed that mitochondria have two membrane systems as outer and inner membranes (fig. 3). Hence, there are two compartments in mitochondria: the intermembrane space between the outer and inner membranes, and the matrix, which is bounded by the inner membrane. Since oxidative phosphorylation takes place in the inner mitochondrial membrane, mitochondria occupy a pivotal position of energy production of the cell. The energy production is exclusively carried out in the mitochondrial electron transport system (complex I, II, III, and IV) together with adenosine triphosphatase (complex V).

Genetic studies led to the discovery of a mtDNA distinct from the nuclear one [28]. The matrix of mitochondria contains two or three copies of mtDNA, and several thousands of mtDNA exist in a cell [29, 30]. Human mtDNA is a double helical circle containing 16,569 bp, which encodes 13 subunits of mitochondrial energy production system, 22 tRNAs, and 2 rRNAs (fig. 4) [31]. For example, complex I consists of 7 subunits encoded in mtDNA and 18 subunits encoded in nuclear DNA.

A striking feature of the human mtDNA is its extreme economy [32]. Nearly every base pair in human mtDNA encodes a protein or RNA product, and some even do double duty in that the last base of one gene serves as the first one of the next gene. The H strand encodes all of the RNAs and protein products except for the one protein and 14 tRNAs that are specified by the L strand [33].

The compact mtDNA is likely to mutate because mtDNA is very simple, not having histones or repairing systems [33], and the exposition to oxygen radicals leaked from the electron transfer system [34]. The mutations, such as point nucleotide mutation or deletion, will cause a defect in the respiratory complexes, leading to decreased energy production in the cell [35]. Moreover, not only this process, mtDNA deletion might impose oxidative stress with consequent peroxidation of membrane lipids [36, 37]. The impaired molecular assembly of the respiratory complexes due to mtDNA mutations will increase the generation of oxygen free readicals in mitochondria, leading to further degeneration of cells [38].

Accumulation of mtDNA Deletion by Human Ovarian Aging

The effect of aging on energy production has attracted much attention, and cumulating evidence indicates a decrease in the activity of mitochondrial oxidative phosphorylation with increasing age [38–41]. As the ovarian aging, its function decreases dramatically during the menopausal period. Then, we have examined the relationship between ovarian aging and the accumulation of mtDNA mutation [42].

mtDNAs extracted from 34 ovarian tissues which were obtained at gynecological surgeries from women ranging in age from a fetus at 22 weeks of gestation to a 77-year-old woman were analyzed qualitatively using the polymerase chain reaction (PCR) method. The amplification of the 5.5-kb mtDNA fragment which codes from ATPase 8 to ND 5 (fig. 4), revealed the abnormal 0.5-kb band only in the ovaries of the older women (fig. 5). The mtDNA mutation of abdominal muscle tissue which was also collected in the same women to compare with the ovarian tissue was detected in all cases, even in the fetus. These results indicated that the deletion of the 5.0-kb mtDNA could occur in muscular tissues even at a very younger age, however, this part of ovarian mtDNA started to delete around the period of menopause. The deletion site was confirmed to be 4,977 bp between ATPase 8 and ND 5 genes by sequencing analysis (see below).

The detection of the ovarian mtDNA deletion in the 34 cases was summarized in table 1. The occurrence rate of ovarian mtDNA deletion increased along the chronological aging step; only 1 woman in 8 had the mtDNA deletion in less than 39-year-old women including the fetus. In cases aged between 40 and 49 years, the deletion was detected in 8 cases of 16, and all women over the age of 50 years had the deletion in their ovaries except 1 case.

The relationship between regularity of menstrual cycles in the women and the detection of mtDNA deletion were also analyzed because the menstrual regularity is indirectly affected by the alteration of hormonal environment at menopausal and postmenopausal periods. Interestingly, the closer relationship between the ovarian mtDNA deletion and menstrual regularity was observed. In the ovaries of 9 postmenopausal women with amenorrhea, the mtDNA deletion was observed in all cases. Ovarian mtDNAs from the 15 women who has regular menstrual cycles showed no deletion in the mtDNA region except 3 cases.

Contribution of mtDNA Mutations to Ovarian Aging

Recently, the relationship between organ aging and mutation of mtDNA were reported in the brain [38], the cardiac muscle [39], and the liver [40]. As described above, we also reported the mtDNA deletion in the ovary and abdominal muscle by aging [42]. Although aging is a highly complex biological process, mtDNA mutations and subsequent segregation of these mutations during life can be important contributory factors to the aging process.

Three different types of mtDNA deletions have been detected (fig. 6) in several degeneration diseases such as mitochondria myopathy [29, 43], Parkinson's disease [38], and Pearson's marrow/pancreas syndrome [44]. The positions of the deletions are located between the directly

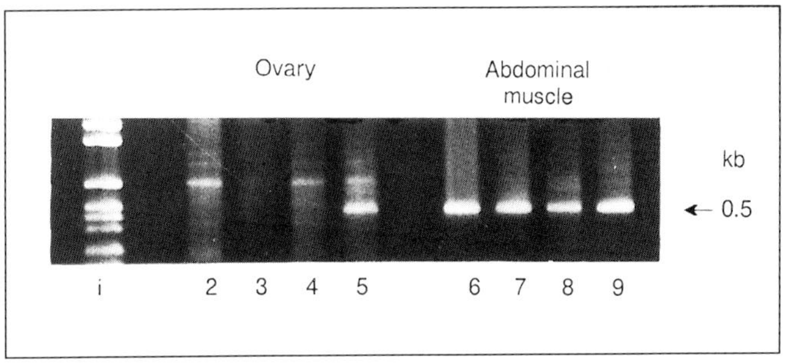

Fig. 5. Detection of the deleted mtDNA in the ovaries and specimens of abdominal muscles. The mtDNA fragments of ovaries (lanes 2–5) and abdominal muscles (lanes 6–9) from a fetus at 22 weeks of gestation (lanes 2 and 6), and women aged 28 (lanes 3 and 7), 45 (lanes 4 and 8), and 77 (lanes 5 and 9) years were amplified by PCR using primers in figure 4. Amplification of the 5.5-kb region resulted in a 0.5-kb band with 5.0 kb deletion of mtDNA in all muscle samples, and ovaries in the postmenopausal woman. The DNA molecular weight is determined with the DNA molecular weight marker (lane 1) indicated 1,230, 1,033, 653, 517, 453, 394, and 298 bp from the top.

Table 1. Detection of ovarian mtDNA deletion related to age and menstrual regularity

Subjects	Cases of mtDNA deletion detected	
	n	%
Age, years		
–29	0/3	0
30–39	1/5	20
40–44	2/9	22
45–49	6/7	86
50–54	5/6	83
+54	4/4	100
Menstrual regularity		
Regular	3/16	19
Irregular	3/6	50
Amenorrhea	9/9	100

Regular: cases who have normal menstrual cycles, including fetus; irregular: cases who had more than two cycles of oligo- and/or polymenorrhea; amenorrhea: cases who have had no menstruations for more than 1 year.

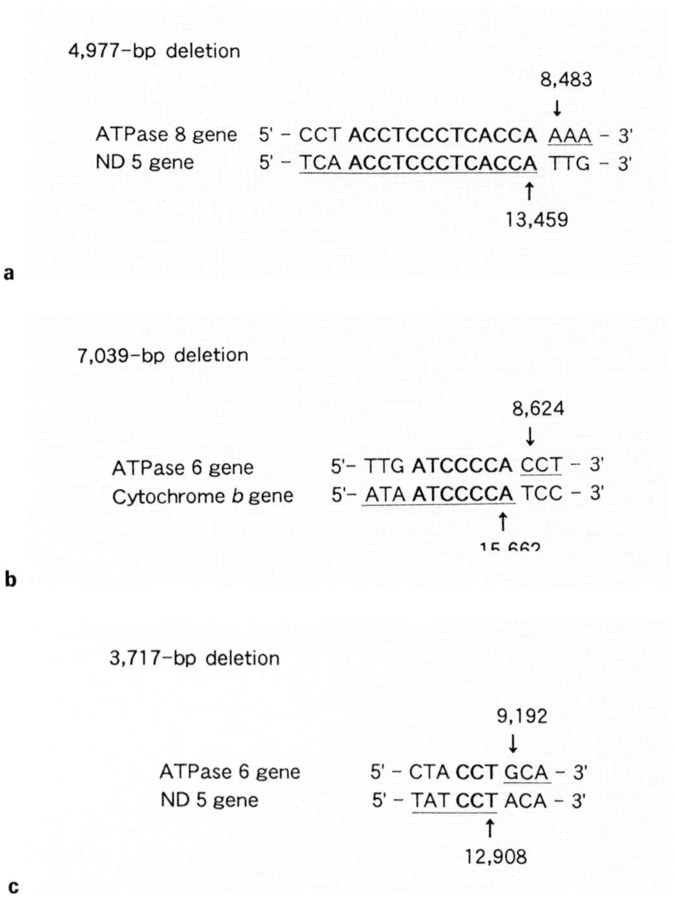

Fig. 6. Deletion patterns of mtDNA. The directly repeated sequences of 13 (ACCTCCCTCACCA), 9 (ATCCCCA), and 3 (CCT) bp are observed in (**a**) 4,977-bp, (**b**) 7,039-bp, and (**c**) 3,717-bp deletion sites, respectively. The numbering of mtDNA are according to the report by Anderson et al. [31]. The 4,977-bp mtDNA deletion (**a**) was not only detected in several degeneration diseases but also in the aged ovary.

repeated sequences present in the mtDNA. The mtDNA deletion of 4,977 bp (fig. 6a) observed in aged ovarian tissues could occur easily because the homologous sequence (ACCTCCCTCACCA) is contained in both ATPase 8 and ND 5 genes [29]. Accumulation of mtDNA deletion of this site is suggested to be linked with not only the pathogenesis of these diseases but also the ovarian aging process.

The deletion of this part in mtDNA spans between the ATPase 8 gene and the ND 5 gene, containing four complex I subunit (ND 3, ND 4L, ND 4, and ND 5) sequences. The decrease in the amount of complex I subunits induced by the mtDNA deletion [45] may cause a decreased energy production similar to a bioenergetic defect in the case of chronic ischemia in the tissue [35].

Although the mtDNA deletion was detected in the ovaries of only menopausal and postmenopausal women, the deletion was observed in the abdominal muscle of all various aged women even in the fetus at 22 weeks of gestation. These observations indicate that the progress of accumulation of mtDNA deletion might vary with different tissues, and mtDNA is kept from the mutation in ovaries of younger women, although the deleted mtDNA rapidly accumulates around the menopausal period.

The analysis of the mtDNA mutation occurrence related to menstrual regularity indicated that the mutation of ovarian mtDNA has a closer relation to ovarian dysfunction by aging. This fact leads us to the following speculations: (1) the accumulation of mtDNA deletion and the resultant decrease of the mtDNA-encoded protein syntheses may affect ovarian function, or (2) ovarian dysfunctions such as the reduced syntheses of steroid hormones with the concomitant increase of pituitary gonadotropin secretions may induce ovarian mtDNA mutation. The data that the mtDNA deletion was detected even in 3 women who had regular menstrual cycles could support the former idea.

The mtDNA deletion in the ovary might be related to the alteration of hormonal circumstances by aging. However, the protection mechanism for ovarian mtDNA mutation in younger women is not clarified. Moreover, the localization of cells where the mtDNA deletion was accumulated could not be determined because the ovary is a heterogeneous organ containing ovum, granulosa, theca, and stroma cells, etc. Further study of these points can evaluate the mechanism of ovarian aging as related to mtDNA mutation more clearly and directly.

In the present paper, we reviewed the human ovarian aging, and the accumulation of mtDNA deletion in the aged ovaries. Since aging should be a very complex physiological process, various factors could be involved for the mechanism of aging. The analysis of these factors will also resolve the clinical problems of menopause and aged women.

References

1 Utian WH, Serr D: The climacteric syndrome; in van Keep PA, Greenblatt R, Albeaux-Fernet F (eds): Consensus on Menopause Research: A Summary of International Opinion. Lancaster, MTP Press, 1976, p 1.

2 Thatcher SS, Naftolin F: Aging and aged ovary. Semin Reprod Encocrinol 1991;9:189–199.

3 Hertig AT: The aging ovary, a preliminary note. J Clin Endocrinol Metab 1944;4:581.

4 Woll E, Herting AT, et al: The ovary in endometrial carcinoma with notes on the morphological history of the aging ovary. Am J Obstet Gynecol 1948;56:617.

5 Bigelow B: Comparison of ovarian and endometrial morphology spanning the menopause. Obstet Gynecol 1958;11:487–513.

6 Boss JH, Scully RE, Wagner KH, Cohen RB: Structural variations in the adult ovary – Clinical significance. Obstet Gynecol 1965;25:747–764.

7 Dennefors BL, Janson PO, Hamberger L, Knutsson F: Hilus cells from human postmenopausal ovaries: Gonadotropin sensitivity, steroid and cyclic AMP production. Acta Obstet Gynecol Scand 1982;61:413–416.

8 Block E: Quantitative morphological investigations of follicular system in women. Variations at different ages. Acta Anat 1952;14:108–123.

9 Baker TG: A quantitative and cytological study of germ cells of human ovaries. Proc R Soc Lond (Biol) 1963;158:417–433.

10 Zuckerman S: The number of oocytes in the mature ovary. Recent Prog Hormone Res 1961;6:63–89.

11 Richardson SJ, Senikas V, Nelson JF: Follicular depletion during the menopausal transition: Evidence for accelerated loss and ultimate exhaustion. J Clin Endocrinol Metab 1987;65: 1231–1237.

12 Dennefors BL, Janson PO, Knutsson F, Hamberger L: Steroid production to gonadotropin in isolated stromal tissue of human postmenopausal ovaries. Am J Obstet Gynecol 1980;136: 997.

13 Fienberg R, Cohen RB: A comparative histochemical study of the ovarian stromal lipid band, stromal theca cell and normal ovarian follicular apparatus. Am J Obstet Gynecol 1965;92:958–969.

14 Mattingly RF, Haung WY: Steroidogenesis of the menopausal and postmenopausal ovary. Am J Obstet Gynecol 1969;103:679–693.

15 Poliak A, Jones GES, Goldberg B, Solomon D, Wooddruff JD: Effect of human chorionic gonadotropin on postmenopausal women. Am J Obstet Gynecol 1968;101:731–739.

16 Judd HL, Judd GE, Lucas WE, Yen SSC: Endocrine function of the postmenopausal ovary: Concentration of androgens and estrogens in ovarian and peripheral vein blood. J Clin Endocrinol Metab 1974;39:1020–1024.

17 Sherman BM, Korenman SG: Hormonal characteristics of the human menstrual cycle throughout reproductive life. J Clin Invest 1975;55:699–706.

18 Yen SCC: The biology of menopause. J Reprod Med 1977;49:287.

19 Sherman BM, West JH, Korenman SG: The menopausal transition; analysis of LH, FSH, estradiol, and progesterone concentrations during menstrual cycles of older women. J Clin Enocrinol Metab 1976;42:629–636.

20 Metcalf MG, Donald RA, Livesey JH: Pituitary-ovarian function before, during and after the menopause: A longitudinal study. Clin Endocrinol 1982;17:489–494.

21 Greenblatt RB, Colle ML, Mahesh VB: Ovarian and adrenal steroid production in the postmenopausal woman. Obstet Gynecol 1976;47: 383–387.

22 Vermeulen A: The hormonal activity of the postmenopausal ovary. J Clin Endocrinol Metab 1976;42:247–253.

23 Poortman J, Thijssen J, Schwart F: Androgen production and conversion to estrogens in normal postmenopausal women and in selected breast cancer patients. J Clin Endocrinol Metab 1973;37:101–109.

24 Tzagoloff A: Mitochondria. New York, Plenum, 1982.

25 Whittaker PA, Danks SM: Mitochondria: Structure, Function, and Assembly. New York, Longman, 1979.

26 Ernster L, Schatz G: Mitochondria: A historical review. J Cell Biol 1981;91:227s–255s.

27 DePierre JW, Ernster L: Enzyme topology of intracellular membranes. Annu Rev Biochem 1977;46:201–262.

28 Attardi G, Borst P, Slonimski PP: Mitochondrial Genes. Cold Spring Harbor, Cold Spring Harbor Laboratory, 1982.

29 Tanaka M, Sato W, Ohno K, Yamamoto T, Ozawa T: Direct sequencing of deleted mitochondrial DNA in myopathic patients. Biochem Biophys Res Commun 1989;164:156–163.

30 Robin ED, Wong R: Mitochondrial DNA molecules and virtual number of mitochondria per cell in mammalian cells. J Cell Physiol 1988; 136:507–513.

31 Anderson S, Bankier AT, Barrell BG, de Bruijin MHL, Coulson AR, Droujin J, Eperom IC, Nierlich DP, Roe BA, Sanger F, Schreier PH, Smith AJH, Standen R, Young IG: Sequence and organization of the human mitochondrial genome. Nature 1981;290:457–465.

32 Borst P, Grivell LA: Small is beautiful – Portrait of a mitochondrial genome. Nature 1981; 290.443–444.

33 Grivell LA: Small, beautiful and essential. Nature 1989;341:569–571.

34 Ames BN: Dietary carcinogens and anticarcinogens. Science 1983;221:1256–1264.

35 Mizuno Y, Suzuki K, Sone N, Saitou T: Inhibition of ATP synthesis by 1-methyl-4-phenylpyridinium ion in isolated mitochondria from mouse brains. Neurosci Lett 1987;81:204–208.

36 Marzden CD: Parkinson's disease. Lancet 1990;i:948–952.

37 Dexter DT, Carter CJ, Wells FR, Javoy-Agid Y, Lees A, Jenner P, Marzden CD: Basal lipid peroxidation in substantia nigra is increased in Parkinson's disease. J Neurochem 1989;52: 381–389.

38 Ikebe S, Tanaka M, Ohno K, Sato W, Hattori K, Kondo T, Mizuno Y, Ozawa T: Increase of deleted mitochondrial DNA in the striatum in Parkinson's disease and senescence. Biochem Biophys Res Commun 1990;170:1044–1048.

39 Hattori K, Tanaka M, Sugiyama S, Obayashi T, Ito T, Satake T, Kanaki Y, Asai J, Nagano M, Ozawa T: Age-dependent increase in deleted mitochondrial DNA in the human heart: Possible contributory factor to presbycardia. Am Heart J 1991;121:1735–1742.

40 Yen T-C, Su J-H, King K-L, Wei Y-H: Ageing-associated 5 kb deletion in human liver mitochondrial DNA. Biochem Biophys Res Commun 1991;178:124–131.

41 Trounce I, Byrne E, Marzuki S: Decline in skeletal muscle mitochondrial respiratory chain function: Possible factor to ageing. Lancet 1989;i:637–639.

42 Kitagawa T, Suganuma N, Nawa A, Kikkawa F, Tanaka M, Ozawa T, Tomoda Y: Rapid accumulation of deleted mitochondrial deoxyribonucleic acid in human postmenopausal ovaries (submitted).

43 Mita S, Rizzuto R, Moraes CT, Shanske S, Arnaudo E, Fabrizi GM, Koga Y, DiMauro S, Schon EA: Recombination via flanking direct repeats is a major cause of large-scale deletions of human mitochondrial DNA. Nucleic Acids Res 1991;18:561–567.

44 Rotig A, Colonna M, Bonnefont JP, Blanche S, Fischer A, Saudubray JM, Munnich A: Mitochondrial DNA deletion in Pearson's marrow/pancreas syndrome. Lancet 1989;i:902–903.

45 Mizuno Y, Ohta S, Tanaka M, Takamiya S, Suzuki K, Sato T, Oya H, Ozawa T, Kagawa Y: Deficiencies in complex I subunits of the respiratory chain in Parkinson's disease. Biochem Biophys Res Commun 1989;163:1450–1455.

Horm Res 1993;39(suppl 1):22–27

Yuji Okatani
Nobuyuki Morioka
Akihiko Wakatsuki
Yuji Nakano
Yusuke Sagara

Department of Obstetrics and Gynecology, Kochi Medical School, Oko, Nankoku, Kochi, Japan

Role of the Free Radical-Scavenger System in Aromatase Activity of the Human Ovary

Key Words
Steroids
Free radical
Aromatase
Estrogen
Ovary

Abstract
The present study was undertaken to clarify the physiological role of the free radical-scavenger system in the control of estrogen production in the human ovary with age. Both superoxide dismutase (SOD) and glutathione peroxidase (GSH-Px) activities in the homogenate of the ovary significantly decreased from the premenopausal period to the menopausal period. The lipid peroxide content, however, showed a small and gradual decrease from the premenopausal to the postmenopausal period. In the premenopausal women, aromatase (Ar) activity in the microsomal fraction of the ovary showed a sharp decline and a significant negative correlation with age. Significant positive correlations were found between SOD and Ar activity, and between GSH-Px and Ar activity. Treatments of homogenate of the ovary with 10, 50 and 100 μM of H_2O_2 resulted in a decrease in Ar activity in a dose-dependent manner. Moreover, treatment with 10 and 50 μM of H_2O_2 produced a more significant decrease in the Ar activity in the premenopausal women than that in the postmenopausal women. Treatments with 0.01, 0.1, 1.0 and 10.0 U of GSH-Px before administration of 50 μM of H_2O_2, on the other hand, induced a recovery of the Ar activity in a dose-dependent manner.

The present study showed the inhibitory effect of peroxide on Ar activity, which was attenuated by GSH-Px. These results seem to suggest that these age-related, relatively free radical predominant environments in the human ovary may have an important role in the decrease of estrogen production through the effects on the Ar activity.

Introduction

The process of aging in the human female is accompanied by characteristic changes in the endocrine system. Among them, a remarkable decline in the production of estrogen in the ovary is the primary feature observed. This decline is consistent with the reduction in ovarian weight and the number of ovarian follicles toward menopause.

Recently, evidence has been accumulating which suggests the existence of a close relationship between the free radical content of certain organs and aging in various animals [1, 2]. The physiological role of the free radical during the process of aging in the human ovary, however, is

Yuji Okatani, MD
Department of Obstetrics and Gynecology
Kochi Medical School
Oko, Nankoku, Kochi 783 (Japan)

0301–0163/93/0397–0022
$2.75/0

still obscure. The present study was, therefore, undertaken to evaluate the age-related changes in the lipid peroxide (LPO) content, superoxide dismutase (SOD) and glutathione peroxide (GSH-Px) activities. The relationship between endogenous LPO and SOD, GSH-Px levels and aromatase activities were evaluated. In vitro studies were also performed to investigate the direct action of peroxide or GSH-Px on the aromatase activity.

Materials and Methods

Preparation of Ovary

Normal ovaries were obtained from 30 patients (36–73 years of age) who received operations for myoma uteri or uterine cervical cancer. Informed consent was obtained from all patients for the use of their ovaries in the present study. In the case of premenopausal women, only ovaries on the early follicular phase of the menstrual cycle (6–8th day) were used. The ovaries were immediately dissected in cold saline and homogenized in 4 volumes of 50 m*M* phosphate buffer containing 0.25 *M* sucrose (pH 7.5), and the homogenate was then centrifuged at 600 *g* for 10 min. A fraction of the supernatant was used for the assay of LPO, SOD, GSH-Px and protein, then the supernatant was centrifuged again at 10,000 *g* for 20 min, and was centrifuged at 105,000 *g* for 60 min and pellet was resuspended in 50 m*M* potassium phosphate buffer containing 0.5 m*M* EDTA, 0.5 m*M* dithiothreitol and 150 m*M* KCl (pH 7.5), and further centrifuged at 105,000 *g* for 60 min. The final pellet of the microsomal fraction was resuspended in 10 m*M* potassium phosphate buffer containing 100 m*M* KCl, 1 m*M* EDTA and 4% (v/v) propylene glycol (pH 7.5) and stored at –80 °C until aromatase and protein assay.

Experimental Protocol

Study 1: Age-Related Changes in the LPO Contents and SOD, GSH-Px and Aromatase Activity. LPO content and SOD and GSH-Px activities in the homogenates and aromatase activity in the microsomal fractions were determined in tissues obtained from 20 premenopausal women (36–52 years of age) and 10 postmenopausal women (51–73 years of age).

Study 2: Effect of H_2O_2 and GSH-Px on Aromatase Activity. Ovarian microsomal fractions from 4 premenopausal women (36–45 years of age) were incubated with 10, 50 and 100 μ*M* of H_2O_2 for 60 min, and used for the aromatase assay. These fractions were preincubated with 0.01, 0.1, 0.5, 1.0 and 10.0 U of GSH-Px for 2 min, followed by 60 min incubation with H_2O_2 (50 μ*M*), and assayed for aromatase activity. H_2O_2 and enzyme were diluted in media. The final volume of the incubation mixture was adjusted to 3.0 ml.

Study 3: Age-Related Effect of H_2O_2 on the Aromatase Activity. Ovarian microsomal fractions from 4 premenopausal women (36–45 years of age) and from 6 perimenopausal women (46–55 years of age) were incubated with 10 or 50 μ*M* of H_2O_2 for 60 min. The incubation procedure was the same as in study 2.

Assay of LPO Content, and SOD and GSH-Px Activity

The LPO content in the homogenates was measured by the thiobarbituric acid (TBA) procedure [9]. GSH-Px activity was determined by the method of Paglia and Valentine [10]. Total SOD activity was determined according to the method of McCord and Fridovich [11]. Estimation of the protein content was based on the method of Lowry et al. [12].

Assay of Aromatase Activity

Microsomal fractions (0.2–0.5 mg protein) containing 3 n*M* 19-[^{14}C]androstenedione (60 μl), 1 μ*M* NADPH, 10 μ*M* glucose-6-phosphate and 1 U glucose-6-phosphate dehydrogenase were incubated in a shaker bath at 37 °C for 60 min in room air. The incubation mixture was adjusted to 3.0 ml with 10 m*M* potassium phosphate buffer containing 100 m*M* KCl, 1 m*M* EDTA and 4% (v/v) propylene glycol. After incubation, chloroform (5 ml) was added to the aliquot (0.5 ml) and the mixture vortexed for 2 min, and then centrifuged at 1,470 *g* for 5 min. A portion of the aqueous layer (100 μl) was taken for scintillation counting to determine the amount of radiolabel released.

Statistical Analysis

Data were expressed as mean ± SD. Difference in the mean values of LPO, SOD, GSH-Px and aromatase were compared by Student's t test. Correlations between aromatase activity and age, LPO content, SOD and GSH-Px activities were compared by regression analysis and the significance of the correlation was estimated by Student's t test.

Results

Age-Related Changes in LPO, SOD and GSH-Px Levels in the Human Ovary

The changes in LPO, SOD and GSH-Px levels in the ovary with aging were evaluated and compared among three age groups: group A comprised 9 women from 36 to 45 years of age: group B 11 women from 46 to 55 years of age, and group C 5 women from 56 to 65 years of age. The mean LPO content decreased with age (fig. 1a). The mean LPO content was significantly ($p < 0.05$) lower in group C (0.526 ± 0.280 n*M*/mg protein) than in group A (0.979 ± 0.466 n*M*/mg protein). However, no significant difference was found in the mean LPO content between group A and group B (0.785 ± 0.217 n*M*/mg protein), nor between group B and group C.

The mean SOD activity showed a significant decrease from group A (6.09 ± 1.57 IU/mg protein) to group B (4.12 ± 1.24 IU/mg protein) ($p < 0.01$) (fig. 1b). However, no significant difference was found in the mean SOD activity between group B and group C (3.62 ± 0.53 IU/mg protein).

The mean GSH-Px activity showed a significant decrease from group A (1.648 ± 0.318 μ*M*/mg protein/min) to group B (1.222 ± 0.287 μ*M*/mg protein/min) ($p < 0.01$), and a further significant decrease was found from group B to group C (0.932 ± 0.180 μ*M*/mg protein/min) ($p < 0.02$) (fig. 1c).

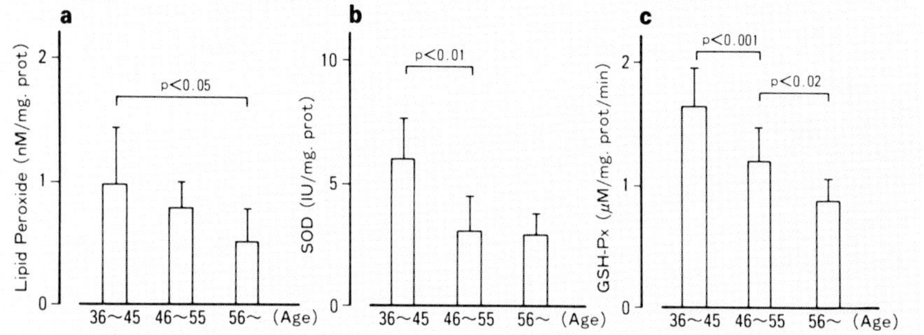

1

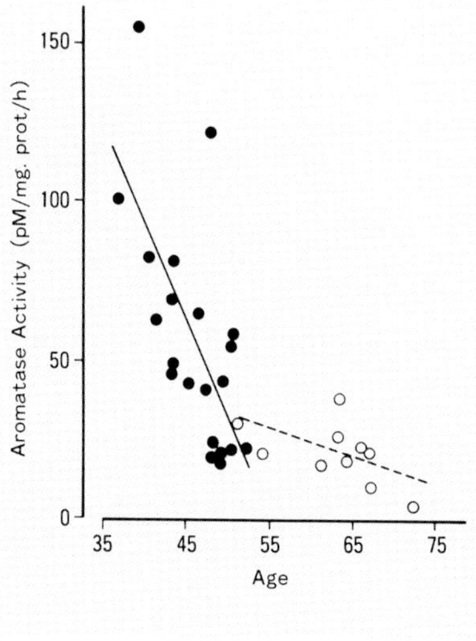

2

Fig. 1. Changes with age in the mean (± SD) values of LPO (**a**), SOD (**b**), and GSH-Px (**c**) in the homogenates of the human ovary.

Fig. 2. Age-related changes in aromatase activity in the microsomal functions of the human ovary. Closed circles indicate the enzyme activity in the premenopausal women, and open circles that in the postmenopausal women. A significant negative correlation was found between aromatase activity and age in the premenopausal women ($r = -0.677$, $p < 0.01$).

Age-Related Changes in the Aromatase Activity in the Microsomal Fraction

Aromatase activity in the microsomal fraction of the premenopausal women showed a sharp decline and a significant negative correlation ($y = -5.793x + 320.5$, $r = -0.677$, $p < 0.01$) with age (fig. 2). After menopause, aromatase activity was low and tended to decrease with age ($y = -0.905x + 77.80$, $r = -0.564$, $p < 0.1$). Furthermore, significant positive correlations were found between aromatase and SOD activities ($y = 15.052x - 1.959$, $r = 0.655$, $p < 0.001$) (fig. 3a), or between aromatase and GSH-Px activities ($y = 37.75x - 0.441$, $r = 0.668$, $p < 0.001$) (fig. 3b). However, no significant correlation was found between aromatase activity and LPO content (figure not shown).

Effect of H_2O_2 on Aromatase Activity

The mean aromatase activity in the vehicle-treated group was 50.5 ± 13.7 p*M*/mg protein/h. Treatment with 10, 50 and 100 μ*M* of H_2O_2 resulted in a decrease in aromatase activity of 89.9 ± 9.0 (n = 4), 55.6 ± 15.3 (n = 4) and 42.9 ± 14.5% (n = 4), respectively, compared to the vehicle-treated group (fig. 4).

Effect of GSH-Px on the Inhibitory Effect of H_2O_2 on Aromatase Activity

The mean aromatase activity after treatment of homogenate of the ovary with 50 μ*M* H_2O_2 was decreased to 43.8 ± 5.8% (n = 4) of the vehicle-treated group. Pretreatment with 0.01 U GSH-Px before H_2O_2 50 μ*M* administration resulted in a mean aromatase activity of 75.3 ± 11.2% of the vehicle-treated group. This value was significantly higher than that in the group treated with H_2O_2 alone ($p < 0.05$). Treatment with 0.1, 1.0 and 10 U of GSH-Px induced a further recovery of the aromatase activity in a dose-dependent manner, being 82.7 ± 3.1 (n = 4), 94.1 ± 4.4 (n = 4) and 107.6 ± 5.7% (n = 4), respectively (fig. 5).

Effect of H_2O_2 on the Aromatase Activity

The mean aromatase activity in the microsomal fraction of premenopausal women treated with 10 and 50 μ*M* of H_2O_2 decreased to 94.0 ± 3.8 and 78.7 ± 7.8% of the vehicle-treated group, respectively. Treatments with 10 and 50 μ*M* of H_2O_2 produced a more significant decrease in the aromatase activity in the premenopausal women than in the postmenopausal women (10 μ*M*: 75.8 ± 10.8%, $p < 0.05$, 50 μ*M*: 47.8 ± 17.5%, $p < 0.01$) (fig. 6).

Discussion

The present study is the first report of age-related alterations in LPO content, SOD and GSH-Px activities in the human ovary. The results show that both LPO content, a parameter of free radical production, and the antioxidant activities of SOD and GSH-Px decrease with age. However, their patterns of decrease are different. Both SOD and GSH-Px activities significantly decreased towards

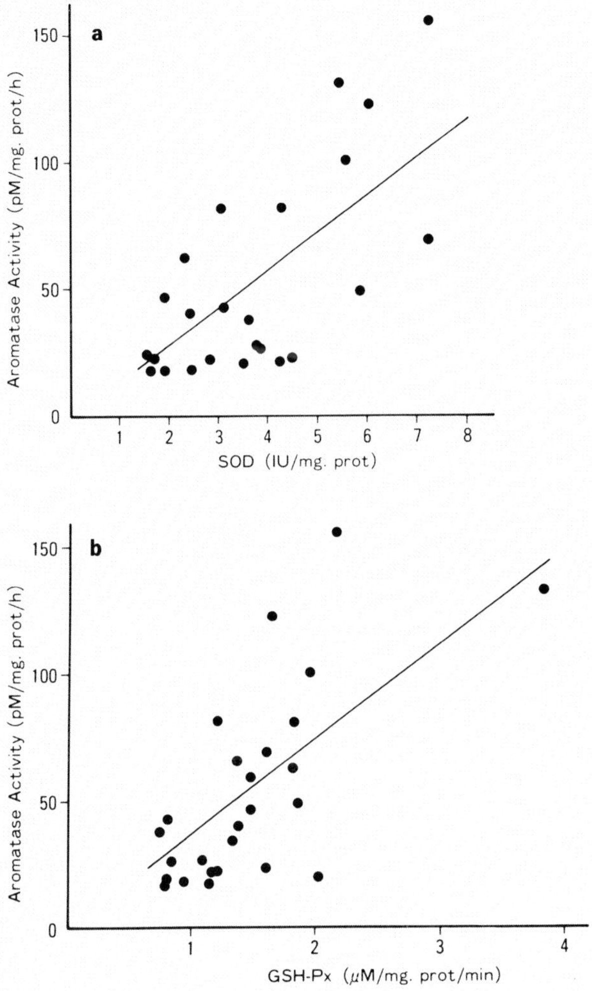

3

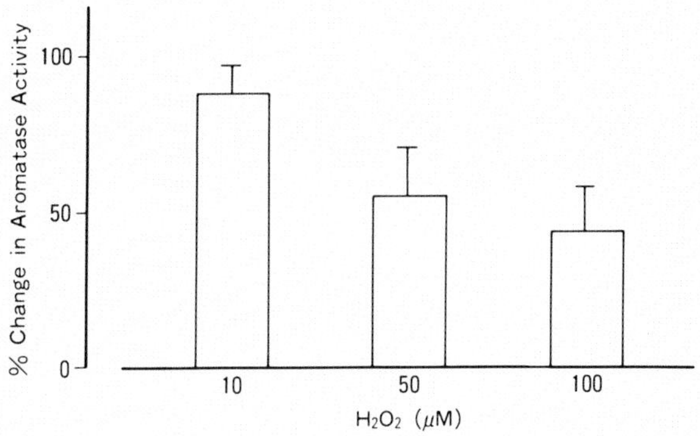

4

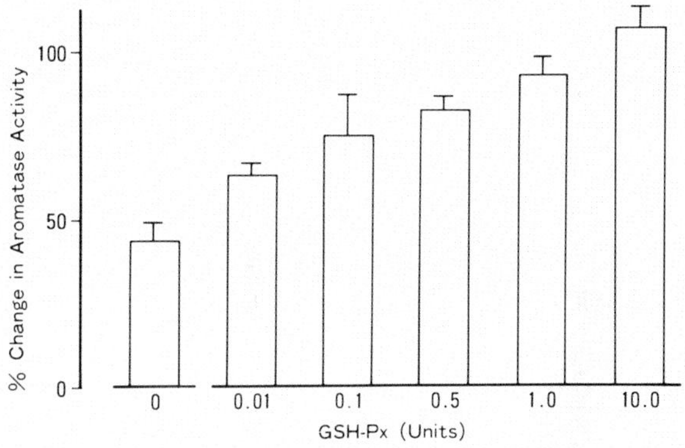

5

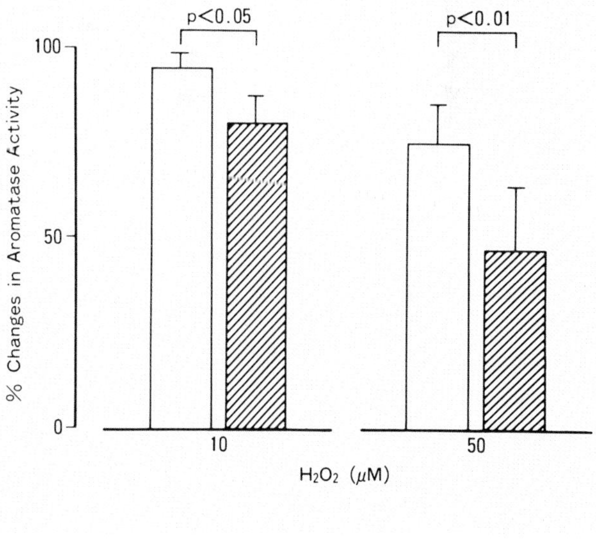

6

Fig. 3. Correlation between SOD and aromatase activities (**a**) and GSH-Px and aromatase activities (**b**) in all the samples from premenopausal and postmenopausal women. Significant positive correlations were found in **a** ($r = 0.655$, $p < 0.001$) and in **b** ($r = 0.668$, $p < 0.001$).

Fig. 4. Dose-dependent effect of H_2O_2 on the aromatase activity. Values are the mean (± SD) percent changes of those treated with vehicle. The microsomal fractions were incubated with H_2O_2.

Fig. 5. Dose-dependent effect of GSH-Px on the H_2O_2 inhibition of aromatase activity. Values are the mean (± SD) percent changes of those treated with vehicle. The microsomal fractions were preincubated with GSH-Px for 2 min, followed by 60 min incubation with H_2O_2 (50 μ*M*).

Fig. 6. Comparison of the effect of H_2O_2 on the microsomal aromatase activity in the premenopausal women (□) and postmenopausal women (▨). Values are the mean (± SD) percent changes of those treated with vehicle. The microsomal fractions were incubated with H_2O_2 (10 and 50 μ*M*) for 60 min.

the menopausal period. GSH-Px activity showed a further decrease after menopause. On the other hand, the LPO content showed a small and gradual decrease from the premenopausal to the postmenopausal period. These patterns apparently indicate that free radical levels progressively acquire a relative predominance over the antioxidative scavenger system in the human ovary with age.

This age-related decrease in the GSH-Px activity has been reported to occur in the liver, kidney and heart of mouse [13], and in bovine lenses [14]. However, as for the changes in SOD activity, the reported results differ with the organs and with the animals studied [15–18]. With regard to LPO, an age-related increase has been reported in the human brain [19], serum and liver of the rat [2], and testis of the mouse [20]. The reason for the characteristic age-related decrease in the LPO content in the human ovary is still poorly understood. Several potential sources of reactive oxygen species have so far been demonstrated within the ovary. Steroidogenesis in response to LH involves oxidation of cholesterol and steroids, and is one of them [8]. Besides, macrophage and neutrophils, evident sources of oxygen radicals, are well documented to reside in both follicles and corpus lutea [21, 22]. Both follicles and corpus lutea are also known to be subject to ischemic episodes, which may also induce the release of oxygen radicals [23]. The remarkable decline in ovarian function towards menopause, which is not observed in other organs, may be related, therefore, to the reduction in the production of oxygen radicals.

Although the activities of most of the enzymes which participate in the production of ovarian steroid hormones decrease with age, the present study confirms the importance of aromatase activity in the decline in estrogen production. The age-related change in aromatase activity is similar to that in urinary estrogen excretions, especially that of 17β-estradiol, which is synthesized mainly by the ovary [24]. These results suggest that the decrease in aromatase activity in the human ovary may be one of the factors in the age-related decline in estrogen production.

It has been suggested that free radicals, by virtue of their chemical reactivity, damage living cells at the DNA level [25], and the cell membrane [26] and other sites as well [27], and that the irreversible portion of this damage is a contributing factor in senescence. Thus, it is possible that the oxidative events play an important role in the changes in enzyme activity. In the present study, no significant correlation was found between endogenous LPO content and aromatase activity, but it should be remembered that aromatase is extremely sensitive to peroxide. The present study showed the direct inhibitory effect of peroxide on aromatase activity. The action of peroxide is rapid and dose-dependent. Moreover, the inhibitory effect of peroxide on aromatase activity is suppressed by treatment with GSH-Px. Furthermore, the antioxidant action of SOD and GSH-Px on aromatase activity was consistent with the finding of significant positive correlations between endogenous SOD and aromatase activities, and between endogenous GSH-Px and aromatase activities. These results indicate that SOD and GSH-Px can exert an antioxidant effect and contribute to protect aromatase activities from the damage of the free radical. This hypothesis is further supported by the fact that the inhibitory effect of peroxide on aromatase activity is smaller in the ovaries from younger premenopausal women, where endogenous SOD and GSH-Px activities are higher, than in those from menopausal women.

The present study revealed a remarkable decline in the activity of the antioxidative scavenger system in the human ovary with age, in contrast to the smaller decrease in free radical production. The results support the assumption that these age-related, relatively free radical predominant environments in the human ovary may cause the decrease in the estrogen production through their effects on the aromatase activity. However, further studies are required to clarify the precise mechanism of the inhibitory action of free radicals on the aromatase activity. In recent years, increasing attention has been directed to the unique antioxidative activity of estrogen [28] and catecholestrogens [29], which are the main metabolites of estrogen [30]. In conjunction with the present results, a remarkable decline in the estrogen production in the ovary may further the reduction of ovarian function with age. However, this thesis requires further study.

References

1 Yoshikawa M, Hirai S: Lipid peroxide formation in the brain of aging rats. J Gerontol 1967; 22:162–165.
2 Takeuchi N, Tanaka F, Katayama Y, Matsumiya K, Yamamura Y: Effects of alpha-tocopherol on thiobarbituric acid reactive substances in serum and hepatic subcellular organelles and lipid metabolism. Exp Gerontol 1976; 11:179–185.
3 Parlow A: Influence on differences in the persistence of luteinizing hormone in blood on their potency in the ovarian ascorbic acid depletion bioassay. Endocrinology 1972;91: 1109–1112.
4 Agrawal O, Galoraya MM: Induction of peroxidase in corpus lutea of rat ovary by lutropin. Biochem J 1977;166:205–208.
5 Laloraya M, Kumar P, Laloraya MM: Changes in the levels of superoxide anion radical and superoxide dismutase during the estrus cycle of *Rattus norvegicus* and induction of superoxide dismutase in rat ovary by lutropin. Biochem Biophys Res Commun 1988;157:146–153.
6 Sawada M, Carlson J: Superoxide radical production in plasma membrane samples from regressing corpora lutea. Can J Physiol Pharmacol 1989;67:465–471.
7 Sawada M, Carlson JC: Association of lipid peroxidation during lutea regression in the rat and natural aging in the rotifer. Exp Gerontol 1985;20:179–186.
8 Chance B, Sies H, Boveris A: Hydroperoxide metabolism in mammalian organs. Physiol Rev 1979;59:527–605.
9 Ohkawa H, Ohishi N, Yagi K: Reaction of linoleic acid by lipoperoxide with thiobarbituric acid. J Lipid Res 1978;19:1053–1057.
10 Paglia DE, Valentine WN: Studies on the quantitative characterization of erythrocyte glutathione peroxidase. J Lab Clin Med 1967;70: 158–169.
11 McCord JM, Fridovich I: Superoxide dismutase: An enzyme function for erythrocuprein. J Biol Chem 1969;244:6049–6055.
12 Lowry OH, Rosebrough NJ, Farr AL, Randall RJ: Protein measurement with the Folin phenol reagent. J Biol Chem 1951;193:265–275.
13 Hazelton GA, Lang CA: Glutathione peroxidase and reductase activities in the aging mouse. Mech Ageing Dev 1984;29:71–81.
14 Chrloff C, Hockwin O, Olson R, Dickman S: Glutathione peroxidase, glutathione reductase and superoxide dismutase in the aging lens. Curr Eye Res 1984;3:109–115.
15 Kellogg EW, Fridovich I: Superoxide dismutase in the rat and mouse as function of age and longevity. J Gerontol 1976;31:405–408.
16 Reiss U, Gershon D: Comparison of cytoplasmic superoxide dismutase in liver, heart and brain of aging rat and mouse. Biochem Biophys Res Commun 1976;73:255–262.
17 Massie HR, Aiello VR, Iodice AA: Changes with age in copper and superoxide dismutase levels in brains of C57BL/6J mice. Mech Ageing Dev 1987;10:93–99.
18 Lammi-Keefe CJ, Swan PB, Hegarty PV: Copper-zinc and manganese superoxide dismutase activities in cardiac and skeletal muscles during aging in male rats. Gerontology 1984;30: 153–158.
19 Chia LS, Thompson JE, Moscarello MA: Changes in lipid phase behaviour in human myelin during maturation and aging. FEBS Lett 1983;157:155–158.
20 Tappel AL, Fletcher B, Deamer D: Effect of antioxidants and nutrients on lipid peroxidation fluorescent products and aging parameters in the mouse. J Gerontol 1973;28:415–424.
21 Cavender J, Murdoch W: Morphological studies of the microcirculatory system of periovulatory ovine follicles. Biol Reprod 1988;39:989–997.
22 Kirsch T, Friedman A, Vogel R, Flickinger G: Macrophages in corpora lutea of mice: Characterization and effects on steroid secretion. Biol Reprod 1981;25:629–638.
23 Marubayashi S, Dohi K, Yamada K, Kawasaki T: Changes in the levels of endogenous coenzyme Q homologes, alpha-tocopherol, and glutathione in rat liver after hepatic ischemia and reperfusion, and the effect of pretreatment with coenzyme Q_{10}. Biochim Biophys Acta 1984; 797:1–9.
24 Sagara Y: The climacteric: Aging of ovary and objective evaluation of climacteric symptoms. Acta Obstet Gynecol Jpn 1989;41:1039–1044.
25 Imlay JA, Linn S: DNA damage and oxygen radical toxicity. Science 1988;240:1302–1309.
26 Girotti AW, Thomas JP: Damaging effects of oxygen radicals on released erythrocyte membranes. Lipid 1984;19:2789–2794.
27 Schraufstatter IU, Hyslop PA, Hinshaw DB, Spragg RG, Sklar LA, Cochrane CG: Hydrogen peroxide-induced injury of cells and its prevention by inhibitors of poly(ADP-ribose)polymerase. Proc Natl Acad Sci USA 1986;83: 4908–4912.
28 Yagi K, Kumura S: Inhibitory effect of female hormones on lipid peroxidation. Biochem Int 1986;13:1051–1055.
29 Nakano M, Sugioka K, Naito I, Taketoshi S, Niki E: Novel and potent biological antioxidants on membrane phospholipid peroxidation: 2-Hydroxyestrone and 2-hydroxyestradiol. Biochem Biophys Res Commun 1987; 142:919–924.
30 Fishman J: Role of 2-hydroxyestrone in estrogen metabolism. J Clin Endocrinol Metab 1963;23:207–210.

Horm Res 1993;39(suppl 1):28–31

Hidekazu Saito
Kazutomo Koike
Takakazu Saito
Makoto Nohara
Shinnosuke Kawagoe
Masahiko Hiroi

Department of Obstetrics and Gynecology, Yamagata University, School of Medicine, Yamagata, Japan

Aging Changes in the Alignment of Chromosomes after Human Chorionic Gonadotropin Stimulation May Be a Possible Cause of Decreased Fertility in Mice

Key Words
Aged oocyte
Alignment of chromosomes

Abstract
The relation between the alignment of chromosomes in the aged oocyte and its capacities of fertilization and development of oocytes was examined. More embryos in the condition of insemination at 12 and 16 h after human chorionic gonadotropin (hCG) however grew into two and more cell stages than those in the insemination of 20, 24 and 28 h. Some embryos in the group of insemination at 12, 16 and 20 h after hCG injection had grown into the blastocyst stage. The embryos inseminated 24 h after hCG and later had shown no further development. Twelve hours after hCG injection, 67% of oocytes have chromosomes on a straight line (A), and 29% have chromosomes scattered in one group (B). Three percent of oocytes have them separated toward both spindle ends (C) and 2% of oocytes have no chromosomes (D). At 16 h after hCG, the alignments of chromosomes are almost the same as that of 12 h after hCG injection. At 20 h after hCG, the most common alignment of chromosomes was scattered in a small group. The alignment of chromosomes of most oocytes was splitting at 24 and 28 h after hCG injection. Thus the oocytes with the chromosome alignment of A or B can be fertilized and developed into the blastocyst stage. The alignment of A and B lasts only about 8 h after ovulation, and the time was extremly restricted for oocytes to develop normally.

Introduction

The primary oocytes remain in dictyotene for at least several years, until puberty is reached. As an individual follicle begins to mature, luteinizing hormone surge starts, and the meiotic division of the oocyte resumes. When fertilization has not taken place, oocytes gradually lose their capacities of fertilization and development. In mice, ova with a postovulatory age of 8 h resulted in fertilization and implantation, but these overripe ova had failed to survive until term [1].

Hidekazu Saito, MD
Department of Obstetrics and Gynecology
Yamagata University School of Medicine
2-2-2 Iida-nishi, Yamagata 990-23 (Japan)

0301–0163/93/0397–0028
$2.75/0

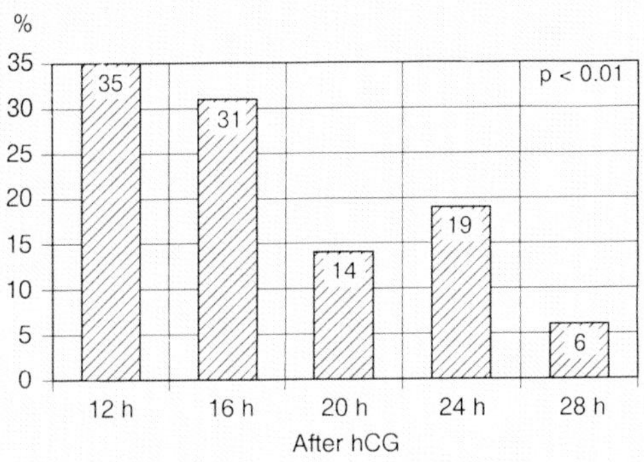

Fig. 1. Rate of oocytes that developed into two and more cell stage 24 h after insemination. There is a significant difference among the groups ($p < 0.01$).

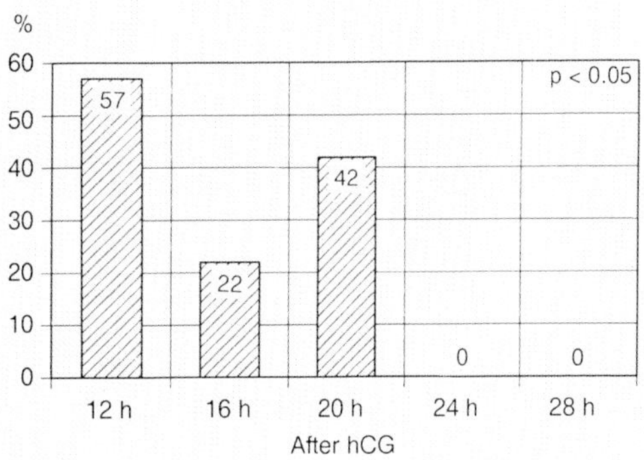

Fig. 2. Rate of oocytes that developed into the blastocyst stage 96 h after insemination. There is a significant difference among the groups ($p < 0.05$).

Meanwhile it has been reported that the chromosomes which are at the metaphase stage of the second meiotic division at the time of ovulation, remain grossly unchanged for about 12 h after ovulation. Eventually a large number of small nuclei form apparently by fragmentation of the chromosome group [2]. Morphological changes in ova during aging are of great interest because various developmental anomalies were attributed to the effects of delayed fertilization [3–5]. In this study, the relation between the alignment of chromosome in the aged oocyte and its capacities of fertilization and development of oocytes was examined.

Materials and Methods

Experiment 1

B6C3F1 mice were stimulated with 10 IU of pregnant mere's serum gonadotropin (PMSG) and 10 IU of human chorionic gonadotropin (hCG). Mice were sacrificed by cervical dislocation every 4 h, starting from 12 h after hCG to 28 h. Oocytes were flushed out of the fallopian tube and washed twice in culture media and then cultured in a culture dish with sperm. A male mouse was sacrificed and the epididymis was put into culture medium and cut by dissecting scissors. Sperms were flowed out from the excurrent ducts into a culture medium. The sperms were then washed twice by centrifugation. One hundred thousand sperms were added to the culture media which contained oocytes. The developed embryos were transferred into a new culture media and then cultured a further 72 h. The stages of embryos (n = 100) were examined under a microscope.

Experiment 2

Oocytes were harvested from fallopian tubes every 4 h starting from 12 to 28 h after hCG. The oocyte-cumulus complexes were incubated for several minutes in the culture medium containing 0.1% (w/v) of hyaluronidase and then aspirated and expirated by a micropipette with a little larger size of inner diameter than the diameter of oocytes. The oocytes were fixed mildly on a glass slide with the medium containing methanol, acetic acid and distilled water (3:1:1). After drying the glass slide was stained with 1% of Giemsa solution. The alignment of chromosomes in oocytes (n = 100) was examined under a phase-contrast microscope.

Results

The oocyte development to two and more cell stages was observed in all the conditions. More embryos in the condition of insemination at 12 and 16 h after hCG however grew into two and more cell stages than those in the insemination of 20, 24 and 28 h (12, 16, 20, 24 and 28 h; 35, 31, 14, 19 and 6%) ($p < 0.01$).

Further development was checked by the formation of blastocyst 102 h after insemination. Some embryos in the group of insemination 12, 16 and 20 h after hCG injection had grown into the blastocyst stage (12, 16 and 20 h; 57, 22 and 42%) ($p < 0.05$). The embryos inseminated 24 h and more after hCG had shown no further development.

The chromosome of five conditions indicated various alignments. Chromosomes are on a straight line (A), are scattered in one group (B), are splitting toward each pole and have split into each pole (C).

Twelve hours after hCG injection, 67% of oocytes have chromosomes in A, and 29% have chromosomes in B. Three percent of oocytes have them in C and 2% of oocytes have no chromosomes (D). At 16 h after hCG, the alignments of chromosomes are almost the same as that of 12 h after hCG injection (A 79%; B 21%; C 0%; D 0%). At 20 h after hCG, the most common alignment of chromosomes was scattered in a small group (A 16%; B 84%; C 0%; D 0%). The alignment of chromosomes of most oocytes was splitting at 24 and 28 h after hCG injection (24 h – A, 20%; B, 15%; C, 61%; D, 3%; 28 h – A, 13%; B, 19%; C, 56%; D, 7%) ($p < 0.01$).

Discussion

The timing of sperm penetration from hCG injection is most important for a female gamete to fertilize and cleave. But in the oocytes, there is apparently a period between normalcy and death. It has been reported that a sperm can fertilize an aging but not yet dead oocyte – such a fertilization could lead to both aneuploidy and polyploidy in animals [6, 7]. In the human there are reports that parents who have an aneuploid offspring often had a different sexual history, i.e. circumstances favoring the possibility of delayed fertilization (contraceptive failure, infrequent intercourse, premarital conception, or religion) [8, 9].

Meanwhile in the case of more aged human oocytes during in vitro fertilization and embryo transfer treatment, for example aged for 2 days, its chromosomes are no longer aligned at the spindle equator but are scattered all over the degenerating spindle and the spindles are pronouncedly shrunk [10, 11]. This implies that human oocytes aged for 2 days may no longer be able to develop into a chromosomally balanced, normal embryo. In the oocytes aged for 3–4 days, typical aging processes such as the migration of the metaphase 2 chromosomes, the more decondensed chromosomes, the formation of a restitution nucleus, and the lagging of chromosomes in the metaphase spindle are observed [10, 13].

The developmental capacity of in vivo- and in vitro-aged oocytes is much lower than freshly ovulated ova [13, 14], and in our data, blastocyst formation was observed in the oocytes aged for 20 h and less after hCG injection (approximately 8 h after ovulation). This implied the development capacity of oocytes was maintained only for less than 8 h after ovulation. Even the oocytes aged for less than 8 h definitely have some incidence of chromosomal abnormality.

The chromosomes of most oocytes aged for 0 and 4 h (12 and 16 h after hCG) were fixed with a straight alignment of the glass slide. The chromosomes in the oocytes aged for 8 h were fixed with one group of scattered chromosomes, because chromosomes may be less tightly stuck to the spindly equator. Most oocytes aged for 12 and 16 h (24 and 28 h after hCG) have chromosomes displaced from the spindle equator towards one of the spindle poles.

These results implied oocytes have a capacity of development as long as their chromosomes are aligned at the spindle equator. The alignment of chromosomes at the equator lasts less than 20 h after hCG administration (less than 8 h after ovulation), and chromosomes then spontaneously displaced towards one of the spindle poles without fertilization, and simultaneously oocytes lost their capacity of embryo development.

Thus the alignment of chromosomes is an important phenomenon to estimate the capacity of oocytes to develop further. Soon after ovulation, the oocytes maintain the ability of development, but if oocytes are aging, and the chromosomes start to move to the spindle poles, oocytes lose their capacity to develop further.

3 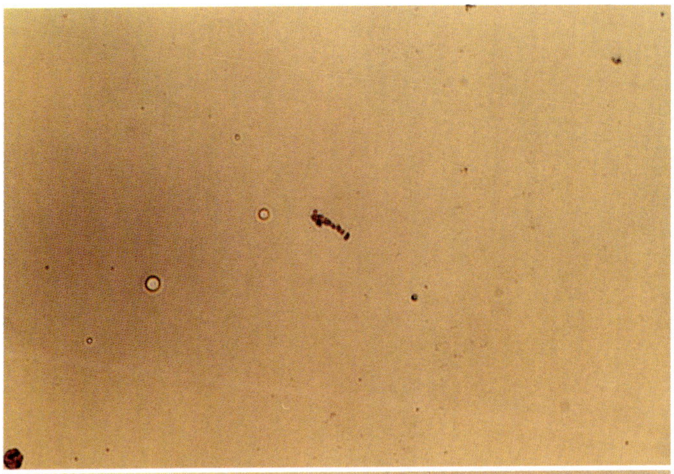 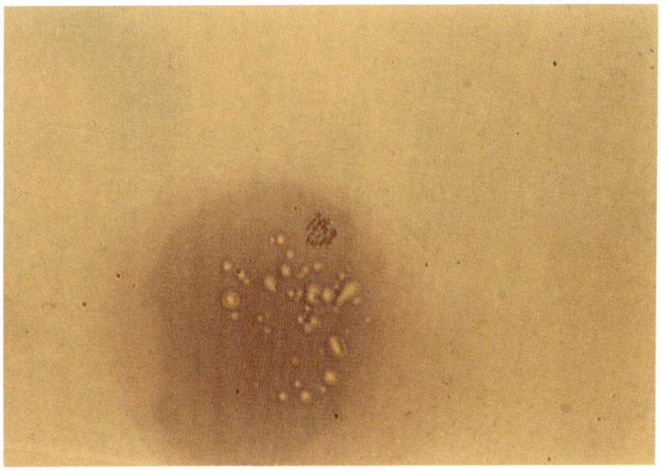 4

5 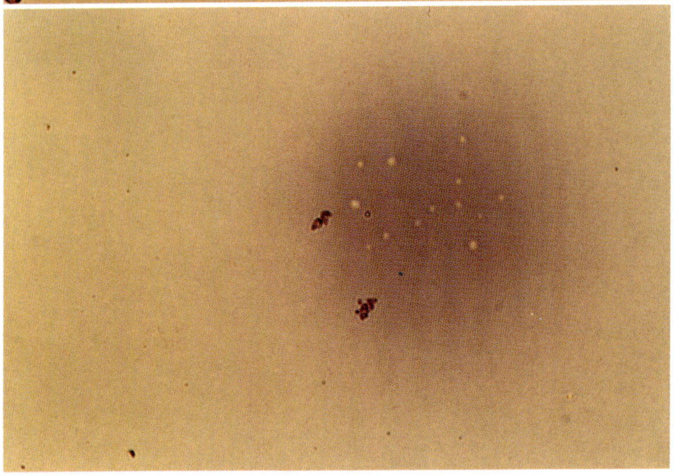

Fig. 3. Chromosomes are aligned in a straight line (A).
Fig. 4. Chromosomes are scattered in a group (B).
Fig. 5. Chromosomes are separated (C).

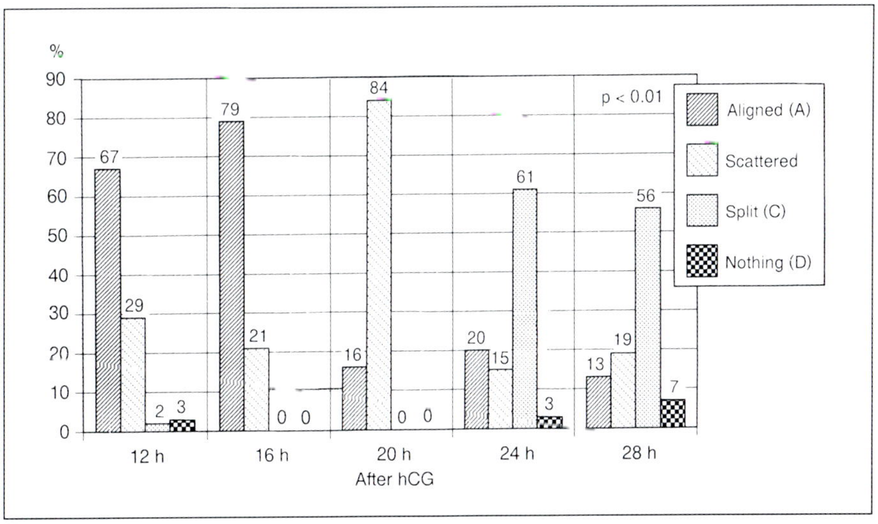

Fig. 6. The rates of various alignments of chromosomes at each age stage of oocytes. There is a significant difference among the groups ($p < 0.01$).

References

1 Runner M, Palm J: Transplantation and survival unfertilized ova of the mouse in relation to post-ovulatory age. J Exp Zool 1953;124: 303–316.

2 Austin CR: Chromosome deterioration in aging eggs of the rabbit. Nature 1967;213: 1018–1019.

3 Austin CR: Aging and reproduction: Post-ovulatory deterioration of the egg. J Reprod Fertil 1970;12(suppl)39–53.

4 Marston JH, Chang MC: The fertilizable life of ova and their morphology following delayed insemination in mature and immature mice. J Exp Zool 1964;155:237–252.

5 Odor DL, Blandau RJ: Incidence of polyspermy in normal and delayed mating in rats of the Wistar strain. Fertil Steril 1956;7:456–457.

6 Lanham JT: Delays during reproduction and their effects on the embryo and fetus. N Engl J Med 1968;278:993–999.

7 Mikamo K, Iffy L: Aging of the ovum. Obstet Gynecol Annu 1974;3:47–99.

8 Juberg RC: Origin of chromosomal abnormalities: Evidence for delayed fertilization in meiotic nondisjunction. Hum Genet 1983;64: 122–127.

9 Sharav T: Aging gametes in relation to incidence, gender, and twinning in Down syndrome. Am J Med Genet 1991;39:116–118.

10 Eichenlaub-Ritter U, Stahl A, Luciani JM: The microtubular cytoskeleton and chromosomes of unfertilized human oocytes aged in vitro. Hum Genet 1988;80:259–264.

11 Eichenlaub-Ritter U, Chandley AC, Gosden RG: Alterations to the microtubular cytoskeleton and increased disorder of chromosome alignment in spontaneously ovulated mouse oocytes aged in vivo: An immunofluorescence study. Chromosoma 1986;94:337–345.

12 Wissen BV, Bomsel-Helmreich O, Debey P, Eisenberg C, Vautier D, Pennehouat G: Fertilization and aging processes in non-divided human oocytes after GnRHa treatment: An analysis of individual oocytes. Hum Reprod 1991; 6:879–884.

13 Gianfortoni JG, Gulyas BJ: The effects of short-term incubation (aging) of mouse oocytes on in vitro fertilization, zona solubility, and embryonic development. Gamete Res 1985; 11:59–68.

14 Juetten J, Bavister BD: Effects of egg aging on in vitro fertilization and first cleavage division in the hamster. Gamete Res 1983;8:219–230.

Horm Res 1993;39(suppl 1):32–36

O. Tsutsumi[a]
Y. Taketani[a]
T. Oka[b]

[a] Department of Obstetrics and Gynecology, Faculty of Medicine, University of Tokyo, Hongo, Bunkyo-ku, Tokyo, Japan;
[b] Laboratory of Molecular and Cellular Biology, NIDDK, National Institute of Health, Bethesda, Md., USA

Evidence for the Involvement of Epidermal Growth Factor in Fertility Decline in Aging Female Mice

Key Words
Aging
Epdermal growth factor
Fertility
Mouse
Ovary
Uterus

Abstract
A decline in fertility, defined as the number of implantat6ion sites, was observed in mice as they aged; the decline started at 30 weeks of age and reached a nadir by 60 weeks when no implantation was detected. Epidermal growth factor (EGF) levels in the submandibular gland and plasma increased as the female mice aged, and sialoadenectomy (surgical removal of the submandibular glands) attenuated the rise in the plasma EGF level without affecting the overall health or survival of the animals. Uterine weight at 10–20 weeks of age was about 70 mg, and it significantly increased with age. This weight has increased more than 2-fold by 60 weeks. These changes closely followed the increase in the concentrations of EGF in the submandibular gland and the plasma. After sialoadenectomy, uterine weight decreased immediately and remained at about 50–60 mg throughout the experimental period. Interestingly, sialoadenectomized mice became pregnant at an older age than the controls. These findings suggest that elevated levels of EGF may have a physiological role in fertility decline in aging mice perhaps via uterine hypertrophy.

Introduction

Fertility decline in the aging females of several species of laboratory animals has been known for many years and is characterized by smaller and less frequent litters [1, 2]. The successful production of litters involves the participation of several organs including the hypothalamus, pituitary, ovary, and the reproductive tract. Failure of any or all of these organs might be responsible for the decrease in fertility. Experiments in mice clearly demonstrated the embryos from older mothers, when transferred to young uteri, survived as well as those from young donors [3, 4], suggesting that uterine aging may be the major cause of fertility decline in this animal. Since steroid hormones and several factors have been shown to control the function of the uterus, it is conceivable that there is one or more growth factor(s) responsible for the decline in fertility.

Epidermal growth factor (EGF), a polypeptide with a molecular weight of 6,045 daltons, is produced in large amounts in the submandibular glands in mice [5, 6]. It is also present in various biological fluids such as the plas-

Dr. Osamu Tsutsumi
Department of Obstetrics and Gynecology
Faculty of Medicine, University of Tokyo
7-3-1, Hongo, Bunkyo-ku
Tokyo 113 (Japan)

0301–0163/93/0397–0032
$2.75/0

ma, urine, and amniotic fluid. EGF receptors are found in various types of mammalian cells, including the uterus [7]. EGF has been shown to stimulate cell proliferation or to modulate cell differentiation in vitro [8]. However, its physiological function has not been well defined. The concentration of EGF in the submandibular glands and plasma increases during gestation [9] and is regulated by estrogen [10]. Estrogen also stimulates uterine EGF production [11].Moreover, EGF deficiency by sialoadenectomy has been reported to cause abortions and intrauterine growth retardation in mice [9, 12], suggesting EGF plays a role in female reproductive function.

In this study we have assessed the fertility decline in aging mice in terms of the number of implantation sites. We also employed sialoadenectomy to evaluate the role of EGF in reproductive function. We found that elevated EGF levels cause uterine hypertrophy, which may be responsible for the fertility decline in mice.

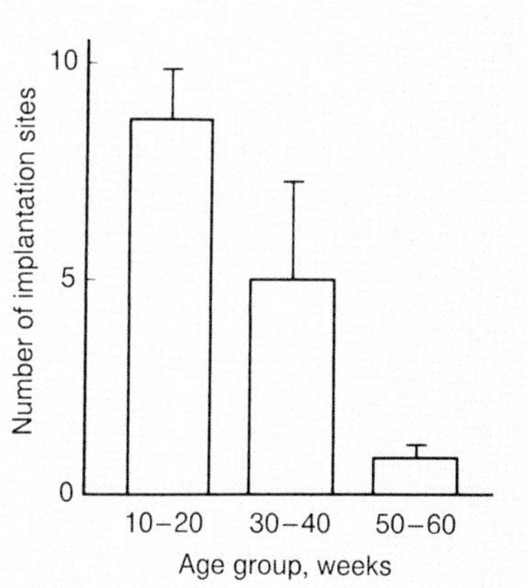

Fig. 1. Number of implantation sites found at autopsy in young and aged mice. Mice with vaginal plug (day 1) were checked on day 7 of their pregnancy. The results are given as mean ± SD. Significant differences were found between the young (10–20-week-old) mice and the old mice by analysis of variance ($p < 0.01$).

Materials and Methods

Female C3H/HeN mice were maintained under controlled temperature (25 °C) and lighting (light from 08:00 to 20:00 h) and had free access to food throughout the experimental period. Sialoadenectomy or sham operation was performed under ether anesthesia when the mice were 7 weeks old. The sham operation consisted of a skin incision and manipulation of the submandibular glands. The animals that underwent surgery recovered quickly without any sign of an abnormality, as judged by general behavior, eating and drinking habits, and weight gain.

Normal and sialoadenectomized mice were sacrificed at various ages between 10 and 60 weeks. Blood was obtained from the trunk vein via a heparinized syringe, and was centrifuged at 2,000 *g* for 5 min at 4 °C. The plasma was aspirated and stored at –80 °C until use. The submandibular glands were excised, weighed and homogenized with 2 ml of ice-chilled phosphate-buffered saline (PBS)/100 mg wet tissue. The homogenates were centrifuged at 12,000 *g* for 20 min at 4 °C. An aliquot of the supernatant was removed and stored at –20 °C until use. The uterus and the ovary were removed and weighed. Te tissue specimens were fixed in 10% (v/v) formaldehyde. They were embedded in paraffin wax and sectioned at 5 µm thickness. Each section was stained with hematoxylin and eosin.

Normal and sialoadenectomized female mice of various ages were mated with mature male mice of proven fertility to assess their fertility. Each female mouse was checked daily, in the morning, for the presence of a vaginal plug, and the day of its detection was designated as day 1 of pregnancy. Pregnant mice were caged individually. In the morning on day 7 of pregnancy, the number of implantation sites was counted.

The EGF concentrations in the submandibular glands and plasma of virgin mice were determined by radioimmunoassay as reported previously [9]. Briefly, 100 µl of submandibular gland extracts, plasma, or unlabeled EGF ranging from 0.01 to 20 ng/assay were mixed with 100 µl of PBS containing ^{125}I-labeled EGF (approximately 15,000 cpm), 1% BSA, and 0.1% sodium azide. One hundred microliters of anti-mouse EGF antisera prepared in rabbits, diluted 1:5,000 with the PBS-bSA buffer containing 1% normal rabbit serum, was then added. The reaction mixture was incubated for 72 h at 4 °C. The antibody-bound EGF was separated from the free EGF by precipitating it with goat anti-rabbit immunoglobulin serum which was diluted 1:15 with the PBS-BSA buffer. Two hundred microliters of the diluted secondary antibody were added to each tube. The reaction mixture was incubated at 4 °C for an additional 24 h. The subsequent precipitate was collected by centrifugation at 8,700 *g* for 5 min and washed 3 times in PBS to remove unbound EGF. The amount of EGF in the precipitate could be determined by counting the amount of ^{125}I-labeled EGF present. The limit of detection of the assay was 0.1 ng/ml, and the intra-assay and inter-assay coefficients of variation were 7.5 and 10.3%, respectively.

The results are given as mean ± SD, and statistical analysis was performed using Student's t test, unless otherwise stated. A value of $p < 0.05$ was assumed to be statistically significant. Mouse EGF (receptor grade) and anti-mouse EGF antiserum were obtained from Collaborative Research, Waltham, Mass., USA, normal rabbit serum from Gibco Laboratories, Grand Island, N.Y., USA, and ^{125}I-EGF from New England Nuclear, UK.

Results

The number of implantation sites on day 7 of pregnancy was 8.8 ± 1.1 in 10- to 20-week-old sham-operated normal mice. There was no difference in the number between the 10- and 20-week groups. The mean number, however, had decreased significantly by 30–40 weeks of age in normal mice and was 5.0 ± 2.2 (fig. 1). Of the mice

Table 1. EGF concentrations in the submandibular gland and plasma of young and aged mice

	Age group, weeks		
	10–20	30–40	50–60
Normal			
Submandibular	49 ± 13	105 ± 17*	194 ± 28*, **
Plasma EGF	0.16 ± 0.06	0.24 ± 0.08*	0.32 ± 0.09*, **
Sialoadenectomized			
Plasma EGF	ND	ND	ND

Results are given as mean ± SD. Each group consisted of 10–15 mice. ND = Not detectable. *, ** Values statistically different ($p < 0.01$) from those obtained 20 and 40 weeks earlier, respectively.

Table 2. Effect of sialoadenectomy on the weight of the uterus and ovary in young and aged mice

	Age group, weeks		
	10–20	30–40	50–60
Uterus, mg			
Control	72 ± 5	113 ± 13⁺	153 ± 20⁺, ⁺⁺
Sialoadenectomized	53 ± 19*	58 ± 17*	64 ± 22*
Ovary, mg			
Control	14.3 ± 1.6	15.2 ± 1.9	12.7 ± 4.7
Sialoadenectomized	14.9 ± 1.8	15.4 ± 2.1	13.5 ± 3.2

Results are given as mean ± SD. * Values statistically different ($p < 0.01$) compared with corresponding control. +, ++ Values statistically different ($p < 0.01$) from those obtained 20 and 40 weeks earlier, respectively.

older than 50 weeks, only a few with a positive plug were pregnant and in these the number of implantation sites was small with an average of less than one. Virtually no implantation site was detected in the 60-week-old normal mice. Sialoadenectomy did not significantly change the number of implantation sites until the mice reached 50 weeks of age. Two out of three sialoadenectomized, 60-week-old mice with a plug had two and three implantation sites, respectively.

The EGF concentrations in the submandibular gland and the plasma in 10- to 20-week-old normal female mice are shown in table 1. The concentrations of EGF in the submandibular gland and the plasma increased with age; the EGF levels in the submandibular gland of the 30- to 40- and 50- to 60-week-old mice were 2- and 4-fold more than those of the younger mice, respectively. The EGF plasma levels also increased by about 50 and 100%, respectively. Sialoadenectomy markedly reduced the EGF content of the plasma and was below the level of sensitivity irrespective of age.

The uterine weight of sham-operated, 10- to 20-week-old normal mice was 72 ± 5 mg. The weight of the uterus increased significantly with age, and it was more than 2-fold greater in the 50- to 60-week-old mice. Histologically, both the endometrium and the myometrium were hypertrophied and the thickness of these two layers was symmetrically increased. In contrast, the uterine weight of sialoadenectomized, 10- to 20-week-old mice was significantly lower by about 25%. The weight gain and the hypertrophy of the uterus observed in the control animals did not occur in the sialoadenectomized mice, and their uterine weight remained about 60 mg throughout the experimental period (table 2).

The weight of the ovaries in the sham-operated, normal mice remained relatively constant at a level of about 14 mg (table 2). Sialoadenectomy did not significantly change the weight of this organ. Histological examination revealed that the number of oocytes significantly decreased wigh age in both the normal and sialoadenectomized mice. A considerable number of developing follicles and corpora lutea were found in the sham-operated, 60-week-old mice (fig. 2a), although no implantation sites were ever observed in those animals with a positive plug. Follicles and corpora lutea were also found in sialoadenectomized, 60-week-old mice (fig. 2b); some had a few implantation sites as mentioned above.

Discussion

The present data showed that fertility decline begins in mice at about 30 weeks of age and they became infertile by 60 weeks. Since a sufficient number of follicles persist in the ovary and ovulation is proceeding at relatively constant rate throughout this period [13], the failure of a blastocyst to implant or of the embryo to develop may be due to defects in the oocyte itself or a failure of the uterus to provide suitable conditions for implantation and embryonic development. Reciprocal transfer of embryos have been made between young (10-week-old) and old

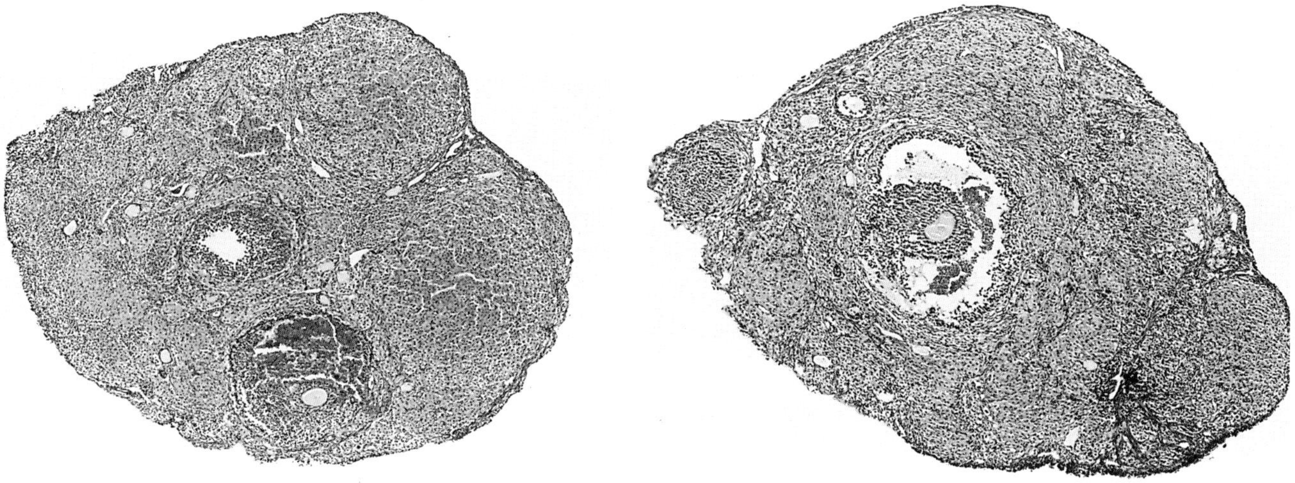

a b

Fig. 2. Presence of follicles and corpora lutea in 60-week-old normal (**a**) and sialoadenectomized (**b**) female mice.

(40-week-old) female mice and indicate that the major cause of infertility is due to aging in the uterus [3, 4]. There is a decline in uterine blood flow as well as a progressive increase in its weight over time [14]. It is difficult to induce a decidual reaction in the aging uterus, which may be due to decreased levels of the estrogen receptor [15, 16]. These morphological and functional changes in aging uterus may be involved in fertility decline.

A significant increase in the submandibular gland and plasma EGF concentrations occurred in female mice between 30 and 40 weeks of age, coinciding with the onset of the fertility decline observed in the animals. The concentration further increased with age. Sialoadenectomy decreased the plasma EGF concentration to undetectable levels and attenuated the increase in EGF levels in aging mice (table 1). These results confirm the previous findings and support the view that the submandibular gland is a major source of plasma EGF in mice [9, 12, 17]. Thus, the possible role of EGF in aging can be studied by performing sialoadenectomies in younger female mice.

The uterine growth in the female mice as they age closely correlated with increases in the submandibular gland and plasma EGF concentrations. Moreover, sialoadenectomy resulted in a decrease in uterine weight and prevented the age-related uterine growth. These results suggest that uterine growth in aging mice is mediated by EGF. Nelson et al. [18] also reported a possible role of EGF in the growth of the uterus. More interestingly, there were some implantation sites in sialoadenectomized, 60-week-old mice without uterine enlargement while there was none in sham-operated mice with enlarged uteri. These results indicate a possible role of EGF in fertility. However, this could not be further assessed because of the limited availability of aged mice and the decreased mating rate in these animals.

Unlike in humans, ovarian activity continues until the latter half of life in mice as reported previously [1, 19] and here. Thus, it is conceivable that the primary cause of reproductive decline is not ovarian aging although the ovary may be affected to some extent by aging. Since estrogen is involved in EGF production in the submandibular gland [10] and the uterus [18], it is also possible that a slight change in ovarian function may limit uterine function. The precise mechanism of fertility decline involving uterine aging remains to be elucidated.

References

1 Finn CA: Investigations into reproductive ageing in experimental animals; in Beard I, Robert J (eds): The Menopause. Lancaster, MTP Press, 1976, pp 1–23.

2 Adams CE: Ageing and reproduction in the female mammal with particular reference to the rabbit. J Reprod Fertil 1970;12:1–16.

3 Talbert GB: Effect of maternal age on postimplantation reproductive failure in mice. J Reprod Fertil 1971;24:449–452.

4 Gosden RG: Survival of transferred C57B1 mouse embryos: Effects of age of donor and recipient. Fertil Steril 1974;25:348–351.

5 Cohen S, Savage CR: Recent studies on the chemistry and biology of epidermal growth factor. Recent Prog Horm Res 1974;30:551–574.

6 Fisher DA: Hormone epidermal growth factor interactions in development. Horm Res 1990; 33:69–75.

7 Mukku VR, Stancel GM: Regulation of epidermal growth factor receptor by estrogen. J Biol Chem 1985;260:9820–9824.

8 Hollenberg MD: Epidermal growth factor – urogastrone, a polypeptide acquiring hormonal status. Vitam Horm 1979;37:69–110.

9 Tsutsumi O, Oka T: Epidermal growth factor deficiency during pregnancy causes abortion in mice. Am J Obstet Gynecol 1987;156:241–244.

10 Kurachi H, Oka T: Regulation of epidermal growth factor by oestrogen in the submandibular gland of female mice. J Endocrinol 1986; 109:221–225.

11 DiAugustine HP, Petrusz P, Bell GI, Brown CF, Korach KS, McLachlan JA, Teng CT: Influence of estrogens on uterine epidermal growth factor precursor protein and messenger ribonucleic acid. Endocrinology 1988;122: 2355–2363.

12 Kamei Y, Tsutsumi O, Kuwabara Y, Taketani Y: Intrauterine growth retardation and fetal losses are caused by epidermal growth factor deficiency in mice. Am J Physiol, in press.

13 Gosden RG: Ovarian support of pregnancy in ageing inbred mice. J Reprod Fertil 1975;42: 423–430.

14 Larson LL, Foote RH: Uterine blood flow in young and aged rabbits. Proc Soc Exp Biol Med 1972;141:67–69.

15 Gesell M, Roth GS: Decrease in rat uterine estrogen receptor during aging: Physio- and immunochemical properties. Endocrinology 1981;109:1502–1508.

16 Chuknyiska RA, Haji M, Foote RH, Roth GS: Age-associated changes in nuclear binding of rat estradiol receptor complexes. Endocrinology 1985;116:547–551.

17 Tsutsumi O, Kurachi H, Oka T: A physiological role of epidermal growth factor in male reproductive function. Science 1986;233:957–977.

18 Nelson KG, Takahashi T, Bossert NL, Walmer DL, McLachlan JA: Epidermal growth factor replaces estrogen in the stimulation of female genital-tract growth and differentiation. Proc Natl Acad Sci USA 1991;88:21–25.

19 Edwards RG: Conception in the Human Female. London, Academic Press, 1980.

Author Index

Numbers refer only to this supplement issue

Subject Index

Numbers refer only to this supplement issue